THERAPISTS' DILEMMAS

Revised edition

Windy Dryden

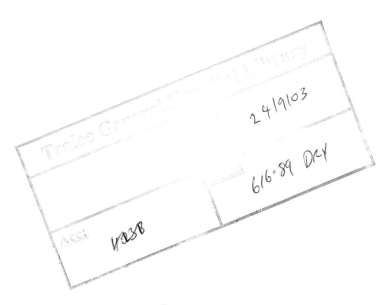

SAGE Publications
London • Thousand Oaks • New Delhi

Chapters 1–15 © Windy Dryden 1985
First published 1985

Chapter 16 © Tim Bond 1997
First published 1997

SAGE Publications Ltd
6 Bonhill Street
London EC2A 4PU

SAGE Publications Inc
2455 Teller Road
Thousand Oaks, California 91320

SAGE Publications India Pvt Ltd
32, M-Block Market
Greater Kailash – I
New Delhi 110 048

British Library Cataloguing in Publication data

A catalogue record for this book is
available from the British Library

ISBN 0 7619 5393 0
ISBN 0 7619 5394 9 (pbk)

Library of Congress catalog record available

Printed in Great Britain by The Cromwell Press Ltd,
Broughton Gifford, Melksham, Wiltshire

To the town and people of Eastbourne

Contents

Acknowledgments

I wish to thank Roz Hussey for transcribing the tapes, my wife, Louise, for typing the first drafts of the interviews, and Michele Markham for typing the final drafts. In particular, I wish to express my gratitude to my colleagues for their participation.

CHAPTER ONE

On the Dilemmas of Being a Therapist

Windy Dryden

Dilemma: A position of doubt or perplexity. A choice between two (or among several) alternatives all of which have some unfavourable elements.

My interest in the topic of therapists' dilemmas emerged a number of years ago when I turned to the research literature for help with a particular dilemma I was experiencing with a client at that time. Unfortunately, my search was in vain. This, however, proved to be fortuitous, since it led me to begin to question the limits of the scientist-practitioner model currently in vogue in the field of clinical practice. Indeed, a perusal of the published psychotherapy literature revealed that therapists rarely discuss their dilemmas in print.[1] And yet therapists do have dilemmas (Morrison, Layton and Newman, 1982[2]), but tend to discuss them *à huis clos*, late at night, over drinks, after formal conference sessions.

In developing the idea for this book, my aim was to attempt to re-create that kind of informal atmosphere where contributors would feel relaxed enough to discuss their dilemmas in public. To achieve this, I decided to use an interview format since this medium most closely approximates the interactive setting in which therapists discuss their dilemmas. I saw my primary task as interviewer as to help the contributors to articulate and explore their dilemmas in a supportive atmosphere. I occasionally asked challenging questions, but in general these were kept to a minimum to preserve the interview's focus on the frame of reference of the contributor rather than to shift it to that of the interviewer.

A comment about the editorial process is appropriate at this stage. Initially, I had each interview transcribed verbatim. Then, I corrected each transcript for grammatical errors and turned it into acceptable English, using a style which reflected the fact that dialogue was being presented. Finally, I invited each contributor to read this 'copy' and to make appropriate changes to style and content. These changes were, without exception, incorporated into the final draft.

What dilemmas do therapists have? Drawing upon those discussed in the following interviews a number of themes emerge.

1. COMPROMISE DILEMMAS

A number of therapists discussed dilemmas which centred on the tension that exists between the 'ideal' and the 'pragmatic'. To what extent should therapists pursue strategies which reflect their ideals, but which flout more practical considerations, rather than sacrifice ideals for pragmatic purposes? Albert Ellis discusses this dilemma in the context of the pros and cons of offering warmth to clients. It emerges in the interview with John Bancroft who confronts this choice whenever he adopts a preferred therapeutic role in cases of sex therapy in which the preferred role may jeopardize successful outcome. Finally, this theme is present in Dougal Mackay's interview in which he discusses being faced with the choice between pursuing conservative (and limited) therapeutic goals, on the one hand, and radical (but more 'risky') goals on the other.

2 BOUNDARY DILEMMAS

The dilemmas with this theme involve the choice of whether or not to cross a variety of boundaries which frame therapeutic work. First, Marcia Davis discusses the dilemma of where to place a boundary around the 'self' in working with vulnerable clients and, consequently, how much therapists should reveal about themselves to such clients with the attendant risks of doing so *and* not doing so. Second, John Davis discusses the boundaries therapists place between their professional and personal commitments and the implications that emerge when the former encroach upon the latter.

Third, Brian Thorne discusses the limitations of traditionally practised psychotherapy from a person-centred perspective and his experiments in devising appropriate therapeutic alternatives. Here, the boundary between appropriate and inappropriate therapist behaviour is particularly salient.

3. DILEMMAS OF ALLEGIANCE

Therapists traditionally turn to professional communities for personal and professional nourishment and support. And yet these communities may also have stunting effects on therapists' ideas about theory and practice. Marvin Goldfried and Fay Fransella both discuss the struggles that emerge when therapists strive to maintain allegiance to a particular school of thought or therapeutic orientation in situations which may conflict with clients' interests. Richard Wessler discusses his experiences on breaking away from a particular professional community and his struggles to establish links with new reference groups.

4. ROLE DILEMMAS

Therapists often encounter much role conflict in the course of their work. John Bancroft discusses the tension he experiences in attempting to move freely between the roles of 'educator' and 'healer' in the practice of sex therapy. Paul Brown articulates his attempts to integrate what he refers to as the 'scientist-practitioner' and 'psychotherapist' parts of himself. While Arnold Lazarus observes that the conditions which satisfy him as a 'clinician' may very well fail to satisfy him as 'researcher'.

5 DILEMMAS OF RESPONSIBILITY

Therapists often struggle with issues of responsibility. In particular, to what degree should they take responsibility for their clients' welfare or to what extent should they respect clients' autonomy and ability to make informed decisions about their own lives? Dougal Mackay discusses this in the context of clinical decision-making and therapeutic involvement of family members. Fay Fransella discusses this issue in the context of her work with a client whose life is at risk.

6. IMPASSE DILEMMAS

Dilemmas relating to responses to therapeutic impasses emerge as the final theme from the interviews. How should therapists respond—when therapy has become stuck—without harming clients but giving due regard to the enduring impasse (Paul Wachtel)? To what extent should therapists make themselves personally vulnerable in their attempts to resolve such impasses (Marcia Davis)? Where should therapists turn when their current state of knowledge is found wanting (Arnold Lazarus)? Finally, and optimistically, in chapter 15 before the concluding chapter, Don Barrister relates his struggle concerning how best to respond therapeutically to the delusional talk of 'psychotics', out of which emerged a relatively successful solution.

This book is not intended for those therapists who are seeking 'cookbook' answers to difficult clinical issues. It is, rather, designed for those who are prepared to be personally confronted by the issues raised in the interviews. To facilitate this process, I have suggested a number of discussion issues at the end of each interview that are pertinent to its content. These are perhaps best discussed in a group setting with open-minded and trusted colleagues.

NOTES

1. Notable exceptions here are: Standal, S. W. and Corsini, R. J. (Eds) (1959) *Critical Incidents in Psychotherapy*, Englewood Cliffs, NJ: Prentice-Hall; and Kopp, S. (1976) *The Naked Therapist*, San Diego, CA: Edits.
2. Morrison, J. K., Layton, B. D. and Newman, J. (1982) Ethical conflict among clinical psychologists and other mental health workers. *Psychological Reports*, 51, 703–714.

CHAPTER TWO

Dilemmas in Giving Warmth or Love to Clients

An interview with Albert Ellis

Albert Ellis is executive director of the Institute for Rational-Emotive Therapy, New York City. He is founder of rational-emotive therapy and grandfather of cognitive-behaviour therapy. He is a fellow of the American Psychological Association, American Sociological Association, American Anthropological Association, etc. He has been president of the Division of Consulting Psychology of the American Psychological Association, president of the Society for the Scientific Study of Sex, vice-president of the American Academy of Psychotherapists, and a member of the board of executives or executive council of several professional organizations, including the American Association of Marital and Family Therapy, the American Asociation of Sex Educators, Counselors and Therapists, and the American Psychological Association.

Albert has published over 500 articles and book chapters and forty-nine books and monographs, including How to Live with a Neurotic *(Wilshire, 1975),* Reason and Emotion in Psychotherapy *(Lyle Stuart, 1962),* The Art and Science of Love *(Lyle Stuart, 1969),* Encyclopedia of Sex Behavior *(Hawthorne, 1967),* Sex Without Guilt *(Wilshire, 1965),* Handbook of Rational-Emotive Therapy *(Springer, 1977),* Theoretical and Empirical Foundations of Rational-Emotive Therapy *(Brooks/Cole, 1979),* A New Guide to Rational Living *(Wilshire, 1975),* A Guide to Personal Happiness *(Wilshire, 1982) and* Rational-Emotive Aproaches to the Problems of Childhood *(Plenum, 1983).*

Albert's main interests are in psychotherapy and sex, love and marital relations, including relationships between therapists and their clients. It is this latter theme that forms the setting for the following interview.

Windy Dryden: Could you put the dilemma that you wish to talk about in your own words.

Albert Ellis: First, it is the dilemma of how warmly to relate to clients in general; and second, how warm to be with very vulnerable clients in particular.

Windy Dryden: Let's take the general case first.

Albert Ellis: I first confronted the general principle years ago when I was questioning orthodox psychoanalytic thought, which holds that early childhood experiences are crucial in determining later disturbance and that clients have to understand and work through these experiences and have a 'corrective emotional experience', as Franz Alexander[1] called it, with an analyst who passively listens to their present and past experiences and feelings.

After seeing that this didn't bring good results, I experimented with Ferenczi's[2] method of active psychoanalysis. He and other people, like Izette de Forrest[3] and Ian Suttie,[4] held that a person's early childhood is even more crucial than Freud thought. Ferenczi claimed that if your parents, and particularly your mother, did not give you enough love, you become emotionally damaged as a result of this lack. Therefore, what an analyst has to be is highly active and really show you the warmth, kindness and love that your parents failed to give you. You will then get that 'corrective emotional experience' and will significantly improve. I experimented with Ferenczi's method in the early 1950s and persisted with it for about a year.

Freud was horrified with Ferenczi's method and said that the next thing Ferenczi would do was to get on the sofa with his clients, particularly with the young attractive females. While I thought Freud's objection was exaggerated, I made sure that the warmth I gave my clients was purely verbal. I didn't touch them at all and I gave verbal warmth to my male and female clients alike.

Accordingly I really went out of my way to tell my clients that they had excellent traits, that I liked them, and that I was sure that they could get over their problems because of their fine traits. I thereby made up for the love they had presumably missed in early childhood. Indeed, many of them actually had been treated unlovingly by their parents. I believed, since I still thought in psychoanalytic terms, that their parents were delinquent and had not given them sufficient love. Since that time I have come to realize that some of these clients were probably obnoxious as children and encouraged their parents' lack of feeling. Also their parents may have been biologically prone to disturbance and may have passed on this tendency to the children genetically.

However, in those days I accepted the hypothesis that these clients were disturbed as a result of lack of parental love, so I gave them a good deal of verbal affection, approval and acclaim. I discovered very quickly that they thoroughly liked this. A good many of them started asking for extra sessions, which they had not asked for before. They also began to show greater warmth towards me and to refer their friends to me for therapy. In addition, I integrated Ferenczi's method with Harry Stack Sullivan's[5] inter-personal approach. I asked my clients about their feelings towards me and talked about my feelings towards them. In talking about my feelings towards them I would include positive appraisals. I did not outrightly lie, but I downplayed my negative feelings towards my clients and emphasized their positive qualities. They loved that!

After six to eight months of conducting therapy in this way, I realized, however, that my clients were becoming unusually dependent on me. In psychoanalysis they became dependent anyway, but with Ferenczi's method they became much more so. I also saw that they were improving very little. Some of them seemed even to be getting sicker, more into themselves and our relationship, rather than involved in their external life.

Windy Dryden: And yet they claimed to be benefitting from therapy.

Albert Ellis: They felt marvellous. They would say such things as: 'I have never felt so good in all my life.' My 'leaven of love' therapy — as Izette de Forrest called it—sometimes helped them feel less depressed, so it was good in that way. However, it didn't help them with their anxiety. They incessantly kept worrying, especially about whether other people loved them. They related well to me and perhaps to a few others. But they didn't improve on their jobs and weren't really doing very well in life. So I started thinking that perhaps this therapeutic method had distinct drawbacks. In fact, as a result of these experiences I first developed the concept which I wrote a paper on years later about clients *feeling* better but not *getting* better. In fact sometimes they got distinctly worse; not all of them, to be sure, but certainly some of them.

Windy Dryden: What was the dilemma at that time for you?

Albert Ellis: The dilemma involved a conflict between therapeutic and practical considerations. On the one hand, these clients were saying how much they were being helped by this warmth method and they were referring many other people to me. Since I was in private practice at that time, and could use their patronage, I knew that if I stopped giving them active approval and acclaim, they would probably drop out of therapy. On the other hand, if I continued in the same vein I would be going against what I felt was therapeutic for them in the long run. So I finally decided to stop giving them so much active approval and some clients did quit fairly soon thereafter. They were no longer getting reinforced, as reinforcement theory would say.

I went on to do a different type of active-directive therapy. I started giving homework assignments and eventually went on to establish RET. Incidentally, the same dilemma arose years later when I had therapists working with me here at the Institute. Some of these therapists seemed to do very well with their clients by using RET *and* a great deal of warmth and affection. The clients liked it and on the surface it looked good. However these therapists often got into trouble with their clients. One therapist in particular got into really hot water because several of his female clients fell madly in love with him. One client bribed the superintendent of his building to let her into his office. The therapist found this client naked on a sofa when he arrived, insisting that he join her because he had led her to believe that he wanted a sex-love affair. He denied that he wanted that, but his warmth towards her had apparently given her this idea. Some of his other clients became overly attached to him and cracked up when he refused to take this relationship further. You see, there is always the danger that some clients will expect more from you, the more warmth you give them.

Anyway, partly for these reasons I formulated RET along less loving lines. But even in RET I have the problem from time to time about how warm to be with exceptionally vulnerable clients.

Windy Dryden: Before we deal with the more specific form of the dilemma, I want to ask you one question. Did these experiences help you to sharpen up your thinking concerning the distinction between short-term and long-term consequences of therapy?

Albert Ellis: Yes. I think so. Because I found that in the short run clients did feel better when I gave them active approval and acclaim. Some apparently made remarkable changes in a brief period of time. However, they usually fell back and didn't continue to improve. I learned from this that short-term warmth is reinforcing and rewarding and will keep people in therapy. That is a big part of the dilemma. A very warm type of therapy will keep clients in treatment for a while—treatment that they could really use. However, if you hook them with this type of approval and they stay in therapy for a year or two, will you then be able to teach them the hard-core RET—namely to think for themselves, to dispute their irrational beliefs, to take risks, and to make themselves *un*comfortable in order later to become comfortable?

Windy Dryden: What has your experience taught you in this respect?

Albert Ellis: My experience is that if you are re lly warm and nice to clients, it leads many of them, as well as yourself, up the garden path because they become dependent on you. When they do finally work at therapy, they do it mainly for you, the therapist — that is, for the wrong reasons. They are not really intent on changing their basic philosophy. They may eventually work at therapy, but usually within their old philosophy, which is frequently a philosophy of 'I need your love.' When they think they need their therapist's love and actually get it they feel good and seemingly improve. But they are not *really* making significant changes.

Windy Dryden: However, if you do not go some way towards satisfying their expectations they drop out of therapy and presumably remain disturbed.

Albert Ellis: That is right. So therefore you had better develop some kind of good rapport with them and show them that you are certainly on their side. The elegant answer to this dilemma is to show clients *un*conditional acceptance. What Ferenczi and his followers really do is to *conditionally* accept their clients. They are implying, 'Because you do good acts and are a nice person, therefore I think you are OK.' However, in RET we practise *un*conditional acceptance and try to show our clients that, no matter how badly they act towards the therapist or towards others, we can still unconditionally accept them and teach them to unconditionally accept themselves. So this is a different kind of acceptance which, when it works, doesn't make clients dependent. In fact, it enables them to become more independent because they become less 'needy'.

Windy Dryden: So these experiences helped you to see that when therapists unconditionally accept their clients this has less dramatic short-term but more therapeutic long-term effects on clients than does undue therapist warmth.

Albert Ellis: Yes. I was also helped to see this at that time by reading Paul Tillich's book, *The Courage to Be.*[6] He clearly encouraged people to have the courage to 'be yourself' and not need the approval of others.

Windy Dryden: OK. Now you mentioned earlier that you still sometimes experience this dilemma, particularly with vulnerable people. Can you elaborate on that?

Albert Ellis: Yes. There are some people who are suicidal and others who are very vulnerable who, if you say anything harsh to them or if you try to push them to do uncomfortable things, just don't seem to be able to take it. So at the beginning of therapy with some people, I lean over backwards to be kinder than I might normally be. I still show them the ABCs of RET and encourage them to do active disputing. But I highlight some of their good traits and push them in the direction of hope. I still have a dilemma because I never know exactly where to draw the line.

This reminds me of the experiences of Maxim Young, who worked in the 1960s at Philadelphia General Hospital, which at that time was a short-stay receiving hospital. Max was using RET with the clients there, some of whom were extremely disturbed. Now Max was very soft sell. He didn't debate or argue with his patients as much as I would do but he was still very educational in his approach to RET. While he reported quite remarkable success with even some of his most disturbed clients, there was one group that he failed to help and who sometimes got worse. These were clients who previously had a very warm therapist who had been very nice to them, who never confronted them, and who strongly complimented them. These clients resisted RET even when taught in Max's toned-down style. They sometimes became more depressed because they couldn't take being even mildly challenged.

I have had similar experiences with clients who also had a very warm therapist for three, five, some even ten years. I have been amazed to discover how little they had progressed during therapy. Yet they spoke enthusiastically about their therapist and told me how much they had learned. However, when I asked them specifically what they had learned, their answers were very vague and they couldn't really point to anything. My experience with these clients yielded more evidence that therapist warmth helps people feel better but tends to leave them far from the point where I would like to see them reach after a reasonable period of therapy.

Windy Dryden: Do you have any instances where you got the balance wrong with these vulnerable clients?

Albert Ellis: Well it's hard to say. I still have a peculiarly perfect record with suicidal clients. I have seen hundreds of them over the years and apparently not one of them has committed suicide while I was treating them and only one or two did so years after they stopped seeing me. I'm warm to most of them at the beginning of therapy because they are very vulnerable. Not all of them are vulnerable, though; some of them are quite hard headed and still suicidal. With the vulnerable ones, however, I combine the warm approach with the RET method of getting straight to the main negative things they are telling themselves: 'I am no good! I will *never* get any happiness! It's hopeless!' I very actively reveal these beliefs and vigorously contradict them. But I tend to do so in a warm fashion. With this approach, I find that many clients get over their suicidal feelings in one, two or three sessions although of course it takes longer to get them over their basic feelings of depression.

However, a number of clients don't continue therapy, perhaps because they think I'm overdoing the warm approach. Some of them tell me to my face: 'Oh you are just saying that because you are a therapist. You don't really like me.' They think I am overly flattering and almost see through what I am trying to do.

Windy Dryden: You seem to be talking about different ways of doing therapy. One type of therapy involves helping clients to get what they want even though this may work against long-term improvement. The other way involves helping clients see, in terms of RET theory, how they are disturbing themselves and how they can get over their disturbance even though this may not coincide with what their own goals are.

Albert Ellis: Well, my own way of doing therapy is to first find out what the client thinks is the problem and start there. I then try to help the client with his or her problem. Then in subsequent sessions I usually check on how the client is feeling, how he or she is using RET, and how homework assignments are being carried out. I usually ask questions such as: 'What

11

bothered you most this week?' or 'What do you want to talk about most?'

The one thing that other RET therapists often do that I rarely do is to ask the question: 'What do you want to get out of this session?' I think that this is an artificial and pressuring question because the client may easily feel compelled to invent a specific goal. If so, therapists will tend to waste therapeutic time by working on the client's goal that they forced him or her to pick. It sounds like a very democratic, consumer-minded thing to do but it often isn't.

The other aspect of therapeutic consumerism that I am sceptical about is when you as the therapist pretend that you and the client are equal collaborators and that you both equally know the answer to the client's problems. This is often nonsense because, when clients bring up a problem, if you are a competent RET practitioner you quickly can guess what they are telling themselves, how to challenge their irrational beliefs and what rational self-statements clients had better produce. So why should you waste therapeutic time collaborating 50-50 with clients when you can effectively help them quickly zero in on what their philosophic problems are—especially their explicit or implicit *musts*. Indeed, if you do try to maintain a fully collaborative stance, I think you are adopting a hypocritical pretence.

Windy Dryden: Why do you think then that therapists like adopting this 'pretence'?

Albert Ellis: My hypothesis is that many therapists, who are scared shitless of making mistakes in therapy, like 'full collaboration' because they can cop out on taking risks and on doing a great deal of the therapeutic work themselves. They are afraid to do active disputing of irrational beliefs and to teach clients how to use the scientific method, which is what good therapy is largely about. They are, in a word, afraid of being directive.

Windy Dryden: Now one criticism that people often make of RET is that you are trying to fit the client to your system as opposed to modifying the system to fit your client.

Albert Ellis: Well, we *are* trying to get the client to fit the system. All therapists do that but many hypocritically deny it. They pretend that they don't use a theoretical Procrustean bed but they really do. Behaviour therapists obviously do and make few bones about it. Rogerian therapists fit clients into their theories about feeling and openness. Gestalt therapists pretend they are spontaneous but of course try to elicit their clients' presumably spontaneous feelings by their own well-planned and highly directive instructions and exercises.

Windy Dryden: And Multimodal therapists?

Albert Ellis: Well, Multimodal therapy overlaps significantly with RET, which was always a multimodal form of therapy a decade and a half before Arnold Lazarus invented his system. Multimodal therapists notably put clients into the BASIC ID system, to make sure they are treated in all these modalties. So what therapists don't fit clients to their particular theory or system? None, I would guess. They all do it, honestly or dishonestly. Remember the research studies which showed that Rogerian therapists reinforce their clients with their 'mm-hmms', even when they are ostensibly is based on that theory?'

Windy Dryden: So what you are unashamedly saying is: 'Yes I do try and fit the client to my theory because I have a good theory and a good therapy that is based on that theory?'

Albert Ellis: Right! I honestly acknowledge that I do. Let's suppose you are a Gestalt therapist and your client says: 'I want to talk about my past.' Or you are a psychoanalyst and your client says: 'I only want to stick to the present. I don't want to talk about my parents.' What do you do?

Windy Dryden: I suppose you have the choice of trying to persuade them to your point of view or referring them on.

Albert Ellis: That's right. If you can't persuade them you refer them elsewhere. So you only stick with your system. Now some systems are more eclectic than others. RET is eclectic in its techniques but not in its theory. It has a theory which states that disturbed people have basic irrationalities, that therapists can identify and can help clients identify very quickly. It also has a theory which holds that to minimize these irrationalities, therapists require many cognitive, emotive and behavioural techniques and not the same ones for each client. Different clients may require different techniques.

Windy Dryden: So again if a client comes in and wants something which you regard as bad for them, you would have no hesitation in trying to talk them out of it.

Albert Ellis: Right. Take for example, hypnosis. I have had my Boards in Clinical Hypnosis for many years and I used hypnosis before I began to practise RET. I have merged RET and hypnotic methods for many years — and so have Don Tosi, Bill Golden and other RET therapists. However, when people ask me for hypnosis I often talk them out of it. Why? Because they have usually read somewhere that it does magic and it will help them enormously with very little work on their part. I therefore try to help them see that this isn't so and try to get them to use RET without hypnosis. However, in certain selected cases, I do combine the two and give them RET within a hypnotic framework.

Windy Dryden: What you seem to be saying is this: 'I am prepared to take the risk and lose clients by not giving them what they ask for, because I often have a clear idea of how they disturb themselves and how they can get over their disturbance and what may sidetrack them from doing this successfully.'

Albert Ellis: Yes. I try to talk them *into* something that I believe on theoretical and practical grounds is therapeutic. I don't always succeed. Some of them go off to other forms of therapy, especially inefficient modes like psychoanalysis. Too bad! But yes, I do take the risk of losing clients because I don't believe in pandering to consumerism in therapy. If I were a grocer, I would hardly sell my customers poisoned food even if they believed that it would magically help them. If I were a physician, I would not give them drugs like amphetamine, even though these might temporarily make them feel better. As a practising therapist I experiment with many techniques, when I think they will work now—and later. But when I have good reason to believe that they will mainly provide temporary relief and do harm later, I do my best to avoid using them. Even when clients whine and beg for their usage!

Let me tell a sad story that epitomizes the dilemma we have been discussing. Over twenty years ago I saw a very healthy 20 year-old woman who was most undisciplined and who had such a dire need for love that she sometimes used a wooden peg leg to get around on (though both her legs were in fine condition) in order to get people to pity her and offer her help.

Although I induced her to use RET to overcome her low frustration tolerance to finally graduate from college, and to finish a novel she intended to write but always avoided working on, I could not induce her to surrender her dire love need. She kept insisting that she would only give it up if I, her therapist, was unusually kind to her and showed that I truly loved her. I stuck to my guns, however, showed her that if I acceded to her demands, I would help confirm her irrational belief that she needed adoration to be happy and self-accepting, and tried to get her to use RET more thoroughly. To no avail. After a year, she quit seeing me and for the next six years saw a psychoanalyst who was very warm to her and gave her the kind of therapy she was certain she needed. When her analyst died, she had a severe breakdown. She married her next analyst, is still a child-wife to him, has never fulfilled her writing or other talents, and still says nasty things to people about me and RET. She keeps sending me carbon copies of letters almost every December showing that she has donated thousands of dollars to various psychoanalytic institutes — and nothing to the Institute for Rational-Emotive Therapy.

Too bad! But I still stubbornly think that I did the right thing by not going along with this client's consumerism and not giving her the love she demanded.

NOTES

1. Alexander, F. and French, T. M. (1946) *Psychoanalytic Therapy: Principles and Application*, New York: Ronald Press.
2. Ferenczi, S. (1952-5) *Selected Papers on Psychoanalysis*, New York: Basic Books.
3. de Forrest, I. (1954) *The Leaven of Love*, New York: Harper.
4. Suttie, I. (1948) *The Origins of Love and Hate*, London: Kegan Paul.
5. Sullivan, H. S. (1953) *Conceptions of Modern Psychiatry*, New York: Norton.
6. Tillich, P. (1953) *The Courage to Be*, New York: Oxford University Press.

DISCUSSION ISSUES

1. *What do you consider to be the role of therapist warmth in psychotherapy?*
2. *What determines how much warmth you show different clients?*
3. *What therapist variables do you think may have short-term value but long-term deleterious*

effects on clients? What impact does making this distinction have on your practice as a therapist?

4. *What do you think are the advantages and disadvantages of 'therapeutic consumerism'?*

5. *Albert Ellis says that all therapists try to fit clients to their own therapeutic system. Would you agree? If so, how do you do this? Do you have any qualms about doing so?*

6. *What approaches and methods do you regard as being harmful for clients? How do you respond to clients who want such approaches and methods?*

CHAPTER THREE

Sex Therapy: Education or Healing?

An interview with John Bancroft

John Bancroft trained in psychiatry at the Maudsley Hospital and was then clinical reader in psychiatry at the University of Oxford from 1969 to 1976. Since then he has been clinical consultant in the Medical Research Council Reproductive Biology Unit in Edinburgh.

He has, throughout his psychiatric career, had an interest in sexual problems and initially was involved in the use of behavioural techniques for the modification of deviant sexual behaviour. This work was described in his first book, Deviant Sexual Behaviour: Modification and Assessment *(Clarendon Press, 1974). Since 1970 he has had a particular interest in sex therapy and has been training people from different disciplines in this form of treatment ever since. He has been instrumental in organizing a training course in sexual counselling in Edinburgh which is now in its fifth year. His current research is mainly into behavioural aspects of reproduction and fertility and in particular the relationship between reproductive hormones and behaviour. He does however have extensive experience in the clinical management of sexual problems of all kinds and has been involved in research in various aspects of human sexuality. He has brought these interests together in his recent book* Human Sexuality and its Problems *(Churchill Livingstone, 1983).*

His principal role is in scientific research and the conflict between his role as a scientist and his role as a therapist is discussed in the following interview.

Windy Dryden: Perhaps you would like to start off by stating the dilemma you experience in your own words.

John Bancroft: There is a conflict between whether I adopt the role of an 'educator' or the role of a 'healer' when I do sex therapy. My preferred philosophy is to help people to learn better ways of relating to one another that they can use in the future. In that sense I see myself as an 'educator'. However, my dilemma is that I may bring about more change, by being the more powerful 'healer'. In terms of my personality it is quite easy for me to present myself as a fairly authoritative figure, and yet in terms of what I think I should be doing, I want to hold myself back in that respect. It may be that some people respond better to one type of approach, and some to the other, I am not sure.

The dilemma is at its clearest at the beginning of a course of counselling with a couple. As the expert 'healer', I would be expected to take a fairly detailed history, get a very comprehensive account of what has gone before in the couple's lives and on the basis of that assessment deliver some sort of authoritative statement as to what I think the cause of their problem is. The type of sex therapy that I use is a modified form of Masters and Johnson's approach and they emphasize implicitly if not explicitly the 'healer' role, by the way they carry out their treatment. For example, they make an authoritative formulation of the case at the beginning of treatment which basically communicates to the couple that the therapists, with their expertise and from a fairly detailed assessment, can see what is the nature of the problem. This authoritative assessment is presented at what they call the round-table discussion with the couple. I feel there is an ethical issue here. I believe that I shouldn't be collecting a lot of very sensitive information from people unless I am clear it is likely to be of some use. Very often one can take a very detailed history and end up not using much of it. But, by then, very confidential material has gone out of the couple's control. I therefore favour a behavioural approach where as you set the couple a series of behavioural assignments so the relevant problems become identified. You can then seek out the background information that you need at the time its relevance becomes clear. But more relevant to my dilemma, I feel that by not taking too comprehensive a history and making too expert an assessment at the beginning of therapy I facilitate the right type of relationship between me and the couple. In other words, they see me as someone they can make use of as an 'educator', someone who will guide them through a new learning experience and who will emphasize that the responsibility for change rests with them rather than with me. In reality I find myself wandering between roles of 'educator' and 'healer' to some extent, not really quite sure where I should be, and I sometimes wonder whether I might get better results if I was more clearly adopting the 'healer' role.

Windy Dryden: So, the 'healer' role is one in which the therapist clearly assesses problems, collects a lot of information, and then makes an authoritative formulation. The healer is the expert, as opposed to the educator who is in a sense more of a guide.

John Bancroft: Yes, but I don't want to oversimplify this. The approach I use is directive and I think it is important to make a distinction between being directive and being authoritative, a distinction which people often confuse. I train marriage guidance counsellors to use sex therapy and they often start off with the expectation that the approach I use is going to be very difficult for them because it is going to be very directive in the sense of telling people how they should run their lives. Well, it isn't like that. However it is directive in the sense of saying: 'These are things that are worth trying. Why don't you try them and let's see what we can learn together from you doing these things. Let's see what you can learn about your own relationship. These are useful things to do. Whether you do them or not is up to you.' In that sense one is directive in doing sex therapy. You start off with a very clearly defined set of behavioural assignments that you ask couples to do. But you use them not simply because they are useful behaviours to carry out, but because they are very effective at bringing into the open the underlying issues. The couple can as a result begin to understand what their basic problems are.

Windy Dryden: And that is what you mean by the 'educator' role?

John Bancroft: Yes, the educator helps the couple to gain understanding of their own and their partner's feelings and helps them to develop new ways of communicating with each other, of dealing with these feelings and so on.

Windy Dryden: So, the educator doesn't say, 'This is what you should do,' but rather, 'You may find these suggestions helpful. If so, fine; if not, let's come back and talk about it and see if we can find a better direction for you.'

John Bancroft: Right. A crucial point is where the couple is left at the end of treatment. If they leave a course of counselling thinking that they have been 'treated' then they are not going to see themselves as being equipped with new resources to deal with problems that may arise in the future. So it is a very important part of my 'educator' role to get the couple, by the time they have left me, to have a clear understanding of what has happened, why it has been helpful, so they can apply these principles themselves. I don't have any conflicts about the 'educator' parts of my role. However, I do have some conflicts about the other parts of my role: to what extent I should be setting myself up as the expert and adopting the mystique of the 'healer'. Quite frequently one or both partners will be looking for that sort of relationship, perhaps because that is what they have learned to expect from helping relationships. Particularly if they see me as a doctor, they may look at me very much in terms of the medical model. So I probably have a greater need to be clearer about this aspect than if I had a different professional background; for example if I was a social worker or a lay counsellor.

Windy Dryden: So, when it comes to the performance of the role of 'educator' you are not in any conflict, you feel comfortable in doing that. The dilemma seems to start when at times you feel that the healing role is more appropriate; does it become more acute when the couple seem to wish you to take this role?

John Bancroft: No, I don't think it necessarily becomes more acute there. If the couple comes into therapy with that sort of expectation, seeking to coax me into the doctor–patient type of relationship—then I would at the appropriate time confront them with this and say that really if they are going to get help from me we will need a different sort of relationship. More of an adult/adult type of relationship, because that is the basis on which this treatment has evolved. Nevertheless, having said that, there are still many ways in which I could be more authoritative. An example of this concerns how I deal with what a dynamic psychotherapist would call interpretations. A crucial part of behavioural psychotherapy is to analyse the difficulties that somebody has in carrying out behavioural assignments. In the course of doing that, you seek understanding of the nature of the difficulty and then look for the appropriate way of resolving it. My dilemma shows itself here in whether I do my best to get the couple to arrive at the correct explanation or interpretation of what is happening themselves, or whether I provide it for them. I tend to work on the assumption, and it's very much an assumption, that it is more effective to get them to come up with the explanation of their own behaviour themselves, rather than have it said from the expert. This is a further example of encouraging the adoption of appropriate problem-solving skills.

Windy Dryden: And yet there is a lingering doubt in your mind whether . . .

John Bancroft: Whether I am too concerned about doing that. And maybe by being more authoritative and saying, 'This is what I believe the reason for your difficulty is. This is therefore what I think you should be doing about it,' I may produce more change in their behaviour.

Windy Dryden: And yet, from what you were saying earlier, you are also concerned about what the couple learn from therapy. You are concerned that they actually take away from therapy skills that they can use to solve future problems. From what you are saying, although the more authoritative type of statement might actually bring about change more effectively in this instance, you would be asking yourself what, however, has this couple learned to help themselves in the future.

John Bancroft: That's right. It is relatively easy to bring about some improvement in sexual problems. The problem is whether the improvement is maintained. You can, simply by reorganizing the behaviour of couples, achieve a reduction in anxiety and an improvement in sexual responses and communciation in that way. This can be enhanced if the couple have developed considerable trust and faith in your ability as a 'healer', when their expectations for improvement are high. You can often bring about quite dramatic improvement in this manner. However, one of the problems that we have in sex therapy is relapse. It is not infrequent to find a couple who improve while they are coming to therapy regularly, but when they stop coming, it is as though the electricity supply has been cut off and they slip back to their original position. It is therefore of crucial importance that they have in their minds some sort of continuing programme that they are going to use after therapy has finished, and, in particular, some clear plan to deal with occasions of failure which are bound to occur. Inoculating people against failure is actually quite an important part of the therapeutic process. In this model I am educating them concerning how to apply the same principles that we have been using during therapy, when future difficulties arise after therapy has finished.

Windy Dryden: You are, then, a professional who is aware of the long-term effects of treatment—in particular, the importance of helping people to develop skills—and you recognize that this is more appropriate to the educator role. Yet you seem reluctant to solve your dilemma by saying: 'The healing role is not an appropriate one for me in this field of work.'

John Bancroft: The dilemma stems from me because I am not sure if I have got it right. All that I have said about being an 'educator' is consistent with my personal philosophy. However I am not sure if I am right in thinking that you actually end up giving people more help by approaching therapy in this way. Therein lies my uncertainty. Whether in fact you might achieve more change, more worthwhile change, by adopting a much more authoritative 'healer' role? That could be one of the explanations for what appears to be a greater superiority of treatment efficacy that Masters and Johnson achieve than other therapists. There are lots of other explanations for those apparent differences, but that is one possibility.

Windy Dryden: So the 'educator' role is consistent with your philosophy. You hypothesize that adopting such a role is going to provide more long-term help for couples because they would have been helped to develop skills that they can use in the future.

John Bancroft: Yes. It may be slower to achieve change but be more durable in its effect. That would be my hypothesis.

Windy Dryden: Yet you have a lingering doubt . . . that this may not be correct and perhaps if you really adopted more of an authoritative position . . . then what would follow?

John Bancroft: Perhaps more people would be helped than at present. Maybe one has to be selective about this and maybe with some couples unless you adopt the 'healer' role you don't achieve very much, while with others the 'educator' role is more appropriate.

Windy Dryden: I wonder if you can say a little more about the sense of reluctance that I am sensing from you about what might be the dilemma for *you* in adopting more of a 'healer' role, more of the time, particularly on those occasions where you feel the educator role isn't being that helpful.

John Bancroft: Well, I suppose some of my reluctance stems from feeling uncomfortable with that sort of status. I am a doctor and I am very conscious and sensitive about how doctors are often perceived. I am also a reasonably strong personality and quite assertive in my relationships with people so that it would not be that difficult for me to adopt that type of powerful 'healer' role in my dealings with people. So I think that at a less conscious or less rational level that explains my reluctance.

Windy Dryden: That you might to some degree be somewhat more assertive and stronger than is necessary?

John Bancroft: Yes. I don't want to be seen in that light. That is not the sort of self-image that I would feel good about. I am very conscious that many other doctors are seen in that light and I don't wish to be identified with them. There are of course certain situations in which it is very important for a doctor to be like that. In times of particular crises, people do need someone with a sense of power, omnipotence even, so that you can turn to them and think that this person is the best doctor in the world for this particular problem and thus invest great faith in them. I think all of us, myself included, probably have a need for that type of person at certain times and therefore I don't decry the medical profession because they are like that some of the time. It's just that I think there are some doctors who find it difficult to be anything else and there are many medical roles—mine would be one of them—where that is seldom appropriate. So again I think this is a particular problem for the medical profession compared with other helping professions.

Windy Dryden: Yet, you have a more personal concern in terms of your self-image and how you would see yourself if you do adopt a more authoritative stance. This seems to underpin a more pragmatic question, namely under what conditions in sex therapy is adopting a more authoritative stance more effective than an educative role?

John Bancroft: Yes. That is a perfectly valid question which deserves a rational answer. I am not sure that we have the evidence to answer it at the moment. I suppose ideally we should be asking that question and seeking research evidence that allows us to answer it. Of course that applies to a lot of other aspects of therapy.

Windy Dryden: It is a valid question, I would agree with you. What you seem to be indicating, and I think this occurs more frequently than therapists actually acknowledge, is that as a therapist you are not free to operationalize that question in that you are not as comfortable in both roles.

John Bancroft: Yes, I think there is another problem for someone like me. I am also a scientist, and have been throughout my career involved in clinical research. I have been involved in a fair number of tightly controlled clinical outcome studies. Basically we are talking about two different hats, to use an analogy—that of the sceptical scientist who tries to avoid making any sort of assumption and that of the healer who requires a certain belief in the correctness of what he is doing in order to convey therapeutic competence. There is therefore a conflict between one's role as a scientist and one's role as a healer. But there is less conflict between wearing the scientist's and the educator's hat, than between the scientist's and the healer's hat.

Windy Dryden: Have you made any attempt to solve this dilemma for yourself?

John Bancroft: No, most of the time I push it to one side and believe that I am right in thinking that I should emphasize the role of educator and yet every now and then I go through phases of doubting this. This occurs perhaps when I have had a particularly unrewarding couple or perhaps when something positive has happened in therapy which seems to be more to do with my being authoritative than being educative. I have quite often thought about it, and when I am training people, I quite often refer to this as one of those things that lingers, and it irritates me that I haven't resolved it yet.

Windy Dryden: So, when you start experiencing the doubt what then? It seems as if you don't just push it to one side, you are able to articulate it, talk about it with other people, but it doesn't seem to change anything.

John Bancroft: Well, it hasn't changed anything very radically.

Windy Dryden: What impact does this dilemma have on your work?

John Bancroft: Well, perhaps hopefully I am going through some sort of incubation process at the moment, without it actually being overtly dealt with. Eventually I hope I will be able to make reasonable and helpful predictions about how I should behave with a particular couple. Perhaps only by having the dilemma in my mind for a reasonable amount of time am I going to be able to arrive at that sort of improvement in the way I work. Perhaps that is the most constructive way of looking at it. But I don't personally believe that I'm going to be able to carry out a piece of research which will resolve that question conclusively.

Windy Dryden: Even if you did do that and got some conclusive data would that necessarily help you freely move between the two roles?

John Bancroft: No, it wouldn't necessarily help. However it could be that if I was reasonably convinced that I was using the 'healer' role appropriately in a particular case I might be more comfortable. Again I don't think it would be difficult for me to behave like that. It's more a question of how I would feel behaving like that. The data would help but not that much.

Windy Dryden: Exactly.

DISCUSSION ISSUES

1. *Would you prefer to adopt the role of 'educator' or the role of 'healer' in psychotherapy? Why?*
2. *To what extent is your self-image implicated in your preferred role?*
3. *When might you emphasize the 'educator' role and when the 'healer' role in therapy?*
4. *If you prefer to adopt an 'educator' role, how do you respond to clients who wish you to be a 'healer' (and vice versa)?*
5. *If empirical research clearly demonstrated the greater effectiveness of your non-preferred role, what impact would this finding have on your therapeutic practice?*

CHAPTER FOUR

To Share or Not to Share? Notes on Myself

An interview with Marcia Davis

Marcia Davis holds a joint appointment as district clinical psychologist for the Coventry Health Authority and as senior lecturer in the psychology department at the University of Warwick.

Her major time commitment is to coordinating and developing the Coventry Clinical Psychology Service and to psychotherapy practice. Working as an NHS clinician in the provinces where therapeutic resources are limited, Marcia is keenly aware of the need for therapy services which offer a flexibility of approach so that a broad range of clients can make use of them. She has also been concerned with the development of supervision and post-qualification training support for clinical psychologists.

Marcia's part-time appointment at Warwick University draws these strands together. She helped establish, together with her husband John, a two-year part-time MSc couse in psychotherapy. This course is designed for qualified clinical psychologists and other professionals who are already practising and wish to further their therapeutic development without being tied to a particular theoretical model.

In her clinical work, Marcia has specialized in relationship problems and psychosexual difficulties. Most recently, she has become increasingly fascinated by the therapeutic issues posed by 'difficult' patients. Challenging and frustrating to work with, she finds they are also often excellent teachers who question the rules of the therapeutic relationship and require self-exploration on the part of the therapist. Not surprisingly, the therapeutic dilemma Marcia has chosen to share is one which arose in her work with such an individual.

27

Windy Dryden: OK, Marcia would you like to put the dilemma that you wish to talk about in your own words?

Marcia Davis: The dilemma that faced me had to do with the issue of confidentiality, although in the case I'd like to discuss it was more focussed on the confidentiality of my own notes about a patient which were detailed and included a lot of material about myself, as well as the patient. Perhaps if I described the case briefly that would be helpful.

This was a man of 31 who had been a school-refuser at the age of 12. He came from a very enmeshed family and managed never to return to school, retiring very much to his own home for the next fourteen years. At the age of 26 he decided that he really needed to venture out into the world and try and make some normal sort of life for himself. He is someone whom one might describe as having rather severe personality difficulties. When I began seeing him there was no contract between us that my notes would be available to him, although I learned later that this had been an issue between him and a social worker he had seen previously. This issue was very much to do with trust. He really was at a rather primitive stage, where the ability to trust and to form a close relationship with another person was still quite an issue. The question of access to my notes about him, which he knew I kept, had several components. Obviously one was to know what I really thought of him and what I really believed about him—could he trust what I actually said, or often what I didn't say because he found a somewhat non-directive style very difficult; silences would feel very hostile to him. Obviously many of the bad negative feelings he had about himself were things which he believed I held about him as well. Although I tried for some time to present his request to see his file in that context it didn't really promote therapeutic movement. We also talked about how much this issue was an obstacle which allowed him to avoid working on other very difficult issues for himself. Mingled with this, too, was his belief that individuals are not accorded proper respect in the Health Service, that patients should have access to their files, to things that are written about them. This is a view that I personally subscribe to. Certainly if I were a patient I would feel that I had a right to know what people had written about me.

Windy Dryden: So, on the one hand, you tried to use his request therapeutically and help him see issues that were underlying his request, yet, on the other hand, you found yourself in sympathy with the surface nature of the request.

Marcia Davis: Yes, that's right. I was also struggling with two other issues. First, if I really wanted him to learn to trust me I also needed to trust him and to trust him with things that were very personal to me as well as to him. Since he was a very difficult person, often hostile, I used my notes quite freely as a way of looking at my counter-transference feelings towards him. So, could I demonstrate that I trusted him? How was he really going to learn about trust while I couldn't trust him and while I remained always in a one-up, somewhat distant position? On the other hand, if I acquiesced to his request, was I also in a way giving in to his difficulty in accepting limits because this was another characteristic of this person—he really did find it hard to accept limits of time and limits of relationship? I think there was one part of him that avoided closeness, because he really feared becoming completely absorbed in a close dependent relationship. So helping him to feel that there were boundaries seemed an important issue on the other side of the fence.

Windy Dryden: So on the one hand how could he learn to trust you if you were not going to trust him? Yet on the other hand in doing so you ran the risk of stepping over a boundary which might have led to other therapeutic problems, those of enmeshment and absorption with you.

Marcia Davis: Another aspect of this dilemma was separating out a personal issue (that if I gave him the notes he had somehow defeated me) from a therapeutic issue (that of helping this man to begin to trust people). How does one tease out one's own needs from the needs of the patient? I also recognized that if he won he might be defeated because he would feel that he had in a way knocked me off my pedestal, and then how could I help him? He located professional people either up on pedestals to be knocked down or as fallen images. If you fail, then you were no good to him. All these issues made it all very entangled for me.

Windy Dryden: So whatever you decided to do could have had a negative therapeutic impact, though for different reasons.

Marcia Davis: Yes. That's right.

Windy Dryden: And there was also the issue of exposing yourself to this particular person. What was your dilemma about doing that?

Marcia Davis: Well, it concerned the very personal nature of my notes as I have indicated before. It really made me come up against myself quite strongly. I really had to decide whether I was prepared to share such personal information with this particular patient.

Windy Dryden: What did you fear that he might do with such information?

Marcia Davis: That was hard to articulate. Looking back I think there was the fear that for him to read such information would undermine the therapy. Also even more vaguely I feared that he might in some sense use it against me with my employers—to suggest possibly that I was not quite competent. His father was a union negotiator, and he tended to present himself in therapy in a confrontational, union negotiating style.

At one stage, although he would not permit me to tape-record our sessions, he brought in his cassette recorder to make his own tapes of me!

Windy Dryden: So you feared that he might use it against you and perhaps harm you professionally, or at least try to?

Marcia Davis: Yes, that's it in a nutshell.

Windy Dryden: Before we go on to look at how you solved this dilemma in terms of what you decided to do, what steps did you take in attempting to reach a solution? Did you engage in much private soul-searching, for example? Did you raise it with other people?

Marcia Davis: Certainly I did a lot of private soul-searching. I also felt quite a need to talk about this with other people. I talked about it primarily with my husband who is also a clinical psychologist. We spent endless evenings after dinner discussing it — the issue would tend to creep into our conversation. I was also aware that I would tend quite anonymously to bring this into discussions whilst I was teaching. Issues which would be discussed on our psychotherapy course would make me think of it and again I might use it as an example. So the dilemma was with me for a very long time and I used several means to deal with it. It was very valuable as a learning experience because it made me confront all kinds of issues about ethics and attitudes which I hadn't personally had to confront before because very few patients had really challenged me to that extent. There are some patients from whom you learn a very great deal, although painfully.

Windy Dryden: So, you made use of your professional community and your professional husband and that helped you to make your decision. What did you decide to do in the end?

Marcia Davis: I decided to let him look at the file, but to protect the confidentiality of other people I removed any letters written to me about him from other people. I arranged for him to come in on a particular day to read the file and then we discussed his feelings about it afterwards. I decided that therapy was not going to move forward if he did not see the file. There was a risk of course that we would not get any further forward because he had seen it but I thought that the lesson that he might learn from my ability to trust him and let him win seemed the most important thing which would come out of it. Some of my colleagues disagreed with that and felt that I was being pushed around by a very awkward person whom they might have discharged from treatment long ago.

Windy Dryden: And that you should have held your ground and said no.

Marcia Davis: Yes. That's right. But I think although there were many good professional arguments and even therapeutic arguments that I could have mustered for saying no, in the end that course of action did not seem the most productive. We would have been struggling over this issue for years without any productive work taking place.

Windy Dryden: Were you tempted to edit your notes or to censor them in any way?

Marcia Davis: I was very tempted to do that. When I read through the notes I saw that I had made some references to him reminding me of some anger I felt towards my teenage son. I also had questioned whether certain things I had said to him were said from a somewhat angry childish position at the time that I said them. However, although I was tempted to edit such matters I decided not to in the end.

Windy Dryden: And what impact did reading your notes have on him?

Marcia Davis: It depressed him at first. Obviously he concentrated a great deal on my account of the sessions. I was holding up a mirror to him and he did not like what he saw about himself. He also expressed a certain amount of anger towards me because I hadn't always been the perfect therapist. He was angry but he also had a sense of vindication that he was right about me. I am not always the perfect therapist. However reading them did help to move him on to face the next issue which had to do with sexuality. This was an issue which he had been struggling very hard to avoid. Our work continued very slowly, but because we had cleared up that issue it became much more apparent to him that it had been a red herring to some extent and that he was partly using it to avoid working on some very personal and difficult issues. Also I think reading the notes helped him to trust me more and feel safer with me. In that sense the experience was quite positive.

Windy Dryden: After that particular episode did you continue to make notes on your sessions with him?

Marcia Davis: Yes. I did.

Windy Dryden: With the same degree of frankness?

Marcia Davis: Now that is a very interesting question. I would say not with quite the same degree of frankness because we had agreed that he could see any further notes that I made. One crucial matter that I probably forgot to mention was that when we were discussing whether he could see my notes I had offered him the chance of seeing my notes from the time we had agreed that they should be made available to him. He rejected this because he obviously wanted to know what I had said about him at a time when I was being completely open and honest, namely before I had agreed to let him see them. I think it is inevitable that when you are writing notes about a patient knowing that he or she is going to see them then you are going to be slightly wary of what you may write. The new Data Protection Bill that will become law is surely going to change the way that we keep our governmental notes.

Windy Dryden: In what way did it affect your note-taking in this particular case?

Marcia Davis: I did not omit any personal reactions, but I was much more circumspect in how I described them. I can't give you a good example of this but I would think twice about my choice of examples and how I phrased my notes. In fact it struck me that if one felt one was writing notes for a patient's benefit one could use it as another therapeutic technique. You could use it as a strategy for inducing further change. So it raised a lot of very interesting thoughts and interesting dilemmas about being open and honest with patients.

Windy Dryden: I guess the next dilemma concerns the publication of this interview?

Marcia Davis: Do you feel that's a worry?

Windy Dryden: Well, to the extent that it involves this person who could possibly read it, who knows. He could say; 'Well look you never asked my permission for this to be published.' Do you take that point?

Marcia Davis: Yes, I take it. I think perhaps I would make a distinction between talking about one's cases where it seems highly unlikely that the person could be identified. I'm using it as an example of a more general issue.

Windy Dryden: Highly unlikely that he might be identified by whom?

Marcia Davis: Obviously, by other people. But if he read this he might think: 'Yes that might be me.' I think that there is a small danger of that, that's right. In that sense maybe I need to get in touch with him to offer him the chance of reading the transcript.

Windy Dryden: And to give his permission or otherwise. OK. Reflecting on that experience, you obviously reread the notes before making your decision. What kind of material might have prompted you to say: 'Well look, such is the nature of my notes that I am really not prepared to take the risk of letting the patient read them even though it might mean that therapy might be stuck on this issue for quite a long time if not for ever?'

Marcia Davis: The whole issue made me realize that my notes are not my exclusive property. They are very much government property and could be subpoenaed and read out in court. Thus one needs to be circumspect not only from the patient's point of view but from one's own. I was glad when I read through them that I did not try to label this patient in any way. I was descriptive of his difficulties, and did not present a theoretical formulation of his problems. Some people could argue that my notes were lacking in this respect. However, I was quite glad I did not do this because I think it helped the patient to see that I saw him as a person and not as a label and that I understood his problems in ways that were also understandable to him. That isn't quite getting at what you asked me, but that's what I would have left out, if I had included it.

Windy Dryden: It seems to me that you were being genuine in the sense that your attitude towards him as a person in therapy was also reflected in the attitude you expressed towards him in your notes. I guess if there was a discrepancy between these two levels . . .

Marcia Davis: That might have been very worrying.

Windy Dryden: On two levels in a sense. First revealing that discrepancy to him and second revealing it to yourself.

Marcia Davis: I think I did express some of my irritation towards him in my writing—irritation which I tried to conceal more in the therapy. Maybe that was a therapeutic error with someone like this. It might have been better if I had directly expressed my feelings of irritation towards him.

Windy Dryden: Did you ask him whether he wished you had expressed some of those feelings that you hadn't expressed in therapy?

Marcia Davis: No, I don't think I asked him that. We did talk more about him realizing that I was human and was not perfect and that one couldn't expect that of a professional. This was the pedestal issue—namely if you are a professional you are setting yourself up to be perfect. It did come out more in that way. It was difficult for me to express my feelings directly to him because I was not entirely sure what they referred to.

Windy Dryden: Returning to the issue which I raised earlier, would there be areas of your own life which you might refer to in your notes which you would not be prepared to show patients even if they asked to see them?

Marcia Davis: I would be quite concerned about revealing sexual areas, although this did not arise with this particular man. Luckily as I get older that seems to be less of a problem for me.

Windy Dryden: Expressions of positive sexual feelings towards a patient?

Marcia Davis: Yes. That might be more difficult to share. I would be very worried about it being very confusing for the patient and also embarrassing and uncomfortable for me.

Another issue is relevant to the general dilemma. When is a patient ready to see these notes, particularly if you haven't written them with the thought in mind that they might see them? It might be quite damaging for patients to read one's notes if they were still in the midst of particularly difficult issues.

Windy Dryden: I guess that raises the dilemma about who actually is the best person to judge whether somebody is ready to receive that information. If it is the therapist then to what extent does therapy become paternalistic?

Marcia Davis: That's right. That was another part of the dilemma that I perhaps haven't brought out sufficiently. Again that's why if you know that your patient is going to read your notes during therapy I am sure you would be much more circumspect about what you write.

Windy Dryden: I can understand that it in fact did make you more circumspect in your note-taking in this particular case. Was this a more general effect?

Marcia Davis: Yes to a degree. However it also made me feel freer to consider the possibilities of sharing notes with patients.

Windy Dryden: Are you raising this issue more with your patients?

Marcia Davis: Yes, especially with patients where I think trust is going to be an issue. Interestingly, often when I bring up the issue, patients aren't bothered. Perhaps the invitation is sufficient for some of them . . . It was generally a growth experience for *me* as a therapist in many ways.

Windy Dryden: Would you have said that while you were in the midst of the situation?

Marcia Davis: I think so. I think it made me realize that one of the excitements of therapy is that it continually stretches me, continually makes me think about my values, my contradictions, my behaviour, my views and the messages I am giving to others.

Windy Dryden: What you are saying then, is really if you had a set policy on this particular issue which you applied to all your patients then you really would not have been confronted with a lot of these issues.

Marcia Davis: Oh, absolutely. If I had just taken a very straight view, and took perhaps a very psychodynamic view, that his request represented resistance which had to be worked through, then yes, there would have been nothing in it for me—just a difficult patient with whom I wasn't getting very far, and that would have been it.

Windy Dryden: So, I guess in a way, we might say that therapists who develop standard policies might do so to some degree for self-protective reasons?

Marcia Davis: Well. It struck me at the time that I wished I was quite rigid about it, because it would have been a lot easier for me and maybe for some of my patients. In a way it is important for many patients to know exactly where they stand and where the boundaries lie. Certainly it can be self-protective because you then don't turn yourself inside out, questioning and trying to sort out what is genuine and what's not.

Windy Dryden: It sounds like it was to some degree a draining experience as you were grappling with some of the issues.

Marcia Davis: Oh certainly. One session with this patient was worth thirty for the rest of the week.

Windy Dryden: Realizing that, did you at the time decide not to take on any more demanding patients?

Marcia Davis: I couldn't say that in all truthfulness because we tend to see patients when they reach the top of our waiting list . . . Perhaps I would take that back. Perhaps that is true. Perhaps at the time I tended to shy away from anyone else who looked as though they were going to be equally demanding. When I finished with this person I experienced both a tremendous relief and also a sense of emptiness because though it was so draining, a challenge had disappeared from my life. I have found others since!

Windy Dryden: So in giving up the painful wrestling you also said goodbye to the challenge.

Marcia Davis: That's right.

Windy Dryden: That's an interesting point on which to end.

DISCUSSION ISSUES

1. *Do you consider that Marcia Davis was being pushed around by a very awkward person or confronted by a fragile individual who had difficulty in trusting another human being? Can you articulate further your viewpoint?*
2. *How might you have responded to this person's request to see his notes? If you decided to let him see them, would you have edited them in any way if they contained personal information about yourself?*
3. *In what circumstances might you let your clients see the notes you had written about their therapy? Under what conditions might you refuse to grant them access?*
4. *What information about yourself are you not prepared to reveal to clients? Why?*
5. *Do you consider that clients have a right to see notes written about them? If so, why? If not, why not?*

CHAPTER FIVE

Commitment: The Price of Keeping Faith

An interview with John Davis

John Davis is currently a senior lecturer in the department of psychology at the University of Warwick. He sees many affinities betweeen his roles as educator and as therapist, and finds the task of establishing productive working alliances with his students, both undergraduate and postgraduate, an absorbing one. Together with his wife, Marcia, he organizes a post-qualification degree course in psychotherapy, the great majority of their trainees being clinical psychologists. In recent years the development and organization of this programme has been the focus of much of his creative energy. He sees the course as providing a mind-expanding experience for course members and hopes that it will ultimately make an impact on the practice of clinical psychology in Britain. He views his aspiration in this respect as akin to a therapist's necessary faith in his capacity as a change agent.

John has always combined his academic work with clinical practice and feels his primary identity to be that of practitioner rather than academic. At present he works sessionally as a clinical psychologist for the Coventry District Health Authority. He is especially attracted to work with so-called difficult patients. In pondering this attraction, he has considered but rejected the notion that it lies in the opportunity to succeed where other therapists have failed. His conclusion, rather, is that these individuals attract him through their capacity to engage, stretch and educate him. As his dilemmas illustrate, they provide him with opportunities to discover himself and his own limits.

In evaluating his achievements, John attaches little importance to his published work. He sees the process of undertaking psychotherapy research as providing a valuable educative experience for the researcher, but is more sceptical about the value of research findings for the practitioner. He is disinclined to share his clinical experience through the medium of writing, preferring an interactive audience; consequently, he finds the prospect of being interviewed about his dilemmas appealing. The achievements from which he takes most satisfaction lie in his contributions to relationships—in his private life, as educator and as therapist. He describes these as the primary sources for his self-regard.

Windy Dryden: OK, John, would you like to put the dilemma that you wish to discuss in your own words?

John Davis: What I would like to talk about is a dilemma involving the commitment I make as a therapist to my patients. The dilemma concerns where to draw the boundaries between my commitment to patients and the commitments I have in my personal life, i.e. to my family and to myself. I thought I might talk about a specific, quite powerful, instance of this dilemma.

Windy Dryden: Perhaps you would like to start with a description of this specific instance?

John Davis: This concerned a young woman whom I first saw several years ago and to whom I became intensely committed. This happened because of the need that she had for my commitment. She was somebody who had very severe problems of trust for reasons which we need not go into here. The particular dilemma arose because she had been involved in a very unpleasant situation where she had for some time been forced to participate in a vice racket. She had extricated herself from it, but during the time that I was seeing her, she was being blackmailed as the price for having run away from the place where she had been working. She was getting herself into quite impossible situations in efforts to find money to meet the demands of her blackmailers. These external problems were making it extremely difficult for her to deal with her basic internal difficulties because she was constantly pressured from the outside. At some point in our contacts and, I guess, probably indirectly with my encouragement, she refused to pay any more money to her blackmailers. One of the consequences of this refusal was that she was brutally attacked by the people involved and was quite badly hurt. I experienced a lot of guilt about this, because in some way I felt partly responsible for it. What also happened after this was that she was warned to discontinue seeing me, because I think the men involved became aware that in some way her contacts with me had been responsible for her refusal to meet their demands. They indicated to her that if I had any sense I would forget about trying to help her with her difficulties, or I might regret it.

Windy Dryden: Was this threat directly communicated to you or through her?

John Davis: No, this came through her. However, I was aware from her of the kinds of action which these people could carry out. I suppose the point at which I became alarmed was when my wife told me that she had received an obscene 'phone-call at home. Although she didn't make much of it, my fantasy was that it was definitely associated with this case that I was working with. I became quite anxious and yet at the same time—this had to do with my sense of commitment and also with issues of confidentiality—I didn't feel that I was in a position where I could breach the confidences that this young woman had given to me. Nor did I feel in any way that I could interrupt the work that I was doing with her. Yet at the same time I felt I was beginning to endanger both myself and my family. So that in a nutshell is the dilemma.

Windy Dryden: So, you felt quite a keen commitment to this woman and even though it looked as if it could jeopardize your own personal safety and that of your family you decided to honour your commitment to your patient?

John Davis: That's right.

Windy Dryden: What on balance helped you to maintain that commitment to her in the face of these dangers?

John Davis: Well, that's an interesting question. I mean, this young woman had such severe problems of trust that it just felt impossible for me to betray the trust which she had placed in me, trust which had taken her some time to develop. She had, for example, previously been in therapy for about a year and a half, and I discovered that she had never been able to share any of the experiences which she had told me about with her previous therapist. When she first came to see me she felt that people like doctors, psychologists, psychotherapists and the like were not to be trusted. Also, perhaps I felt that once I had made a commitment to her, I could not back out of that commitment.

Windy Dryden: So it sounds as if there was a combination of factors there. First there was the question of the severity of this woman's problems of trust; you felt that you could not let her down given the nature of her problems. Second was your sense of responsibility, namely that once you made a commitment you just weren't going to back out of it even in the face of apparent dangers to yourself and your family.

John Davis: Yes. I think that's right. It was a difficult situation because I didn't want to alarm my wife by telling her what was in my mind about the 'phone-call she had received. On the other hand the idea that I might put a commitment to a patient before a commitment to my family was a very difficult one for me to contemplate.

Windy Dryden: And yet that is in fact what you were doing?

John Davis: I think in a sense that is right. There were other aspects to the dilemma as well. I was well aware from what this young woman had told me that were some action to be taken to prevent the operation of this vice racket a lot of other people might also be saved from a great deal of harm. Yet it would have been a complete betrayal of her trust if I had tried independently to inform the authorities about it or take any action of that kind.

Windy Dryden: Did taking that course of action occur to you?

John Davis: Well, I think I recognized that that was a possibility. I don't think I was ever tempted to do it. On the other hand, I did put to her the possibility that the only way for her to escape or put an end to the situation would be to involve the police.

Windy Dryden: Was the 'phone -call the worst that actually happened to you and your family?

John Davis: Yes, in fact my anxieties were never realized, in the sense that nothing else actually transpired.

Windy Dryden: How do you think you would have responded if some of those fears had been realized? If actual threats had been made or actions against yourself and your family had been taken?

John Davis: That's an interesting question. I don't think I had really thought it through. For a period of time what was uppermost in my mind was how I might defend myself if I encountered any difficulties; I was in that sense prepared for some kind of trouble. But ultimately I don't know what I would have done; the rational part of me said it would not be worth the while of these people to invite trouble from somebody in a professional position. But the dilemma was still there in the sense that I didn't know at the time how ultimately I would act.

Windy Dryden: So the limits of your commitment to a disturbed patient that you sensed had a very real need of you were being tested. You were the first person that she had really opened herself up to and just how far were you going to stick to that commitment in the face of real evidence, not just fantasy, but real evidence of danger to your family?

John Davis: That's right. I don't think I have an answer to the question. The question is there. Ordinarily it is not brought out because commitments tend to be self-limiting in some fashion. But one doesn't know what is going to be asked of one in the way of commitment. Perhaps there are going to be occasions when a great deal is going to be asked. I imagine that every therapist has to find out somewhere along the line what the limits of his or her commitment are.

Windy Dryden: Were there any other experiences with this patient that tested the boundary you place between your commitment to patients and your commitment to your family?

John Davis: Yes, I think one or two other instances come to mind. One would be that there were phases when she would be going through acute crises of one kind or another. I would receive crisis calls from her late at night, or at other inopportune times, which involved my going out to see her. My general response to these calls would be to go. On the other hand, I was well aware that this actually created some strain in terms of my family commitments. This patient was taking me away from my family when I would normally be spending time with my children and with my wife at home. And yet I decided to respond to the needs of the patient. So this would be another example of the same dilemma and again one in which at those times I seemed to be putting the needs of the patient before the needs of the family.

Another example with this young woman would be that there were times when I was aware that on leaving a therapy session she would not be able to go home and indeed would have nowhere to go. My dilemma at those times was should I simply let her go knowing that she would spend the night on a park bench or some such place or should I take her to my own home and give her a bed. There were times when I have done exactly that, taken her home and given her a bed in my house. Again that is an intrusion on my own family life. So here again was the dilemma about my commitment to the patient and my commitment to the family.

Windy Dryden: What was the family's response to your decision to place, at times and in these ways, this woman's needs above theirs?

John Davis: Well, I suppose the main person who might be expected to have a say in what I was doing would be my wife, who was really very good about it. She is a therapist herself and understood the issues involved. This didn't prevent her feeling aggrieved at times: 'Oh, not again,' 'You are not having to go out again tonight.' I can recall one occasion when we had some members of my family and other people spending the weekend with us when an emergency arose on a particular evening and again I decided to go out to the patient. Although I am describing these as dilemmas, I don't think in the situation that I hesitated about which way I was going to act. Nevertheless the dilemma existed. There was a source of stress within my family as a result, although not a severe one because the family relationships are good.

Windy Dryden: It sounds as if your dilemma did not concern how you would cope with an acute reaction on the part of your family because apart from moments of feeling aggrieved, your family, mainly your wife, took an understanding and an empathic reaction to it. Your dilemma centred more on the question: should you actually impose on your family in this way? way?

John Davis: I think that's right. I think I experienced quite a lot of guilt about putting the patient before my family. Also there was another issue concerning what is appropriate behaviour for a therapist. I was well aware that many therapists would feel that my behaviour in this case was not an appropriate way for a therapist to act. A therapist ought not to be behaving in this way with a patient.

Windy Dryden: A therapist shouldn't go out and answer calls of crisis, and certainly not invite patients to have a bed for a night?

John Davis: Yes, I could well imagine some therapists looking at me and saying: 'Here is a therapist who has no idea where boundaries belong in his therapy.'

Windy Dryden: How would you answer these criticisms?

John Davis: I don't feel in too much doubt about it myself. I feel that maintaining this bond of trust in this therapy was absolutely critical. I know how easy it would have been to lose the trust that the patient had invested in me. I was very moved by the desperate situation in which this young woman found herself. I suppose she was an unusual patient in that she was able to articulate her inner experience in a very expressive way, she could communicate very clearly how she was experiencing the situations in which she found herself. Perhaps less articulate patients wouldn't have drawn such a strong commitment from me.

Windy Dryden: So you seem to be saying that there was something about this patient that moved you, that touched you in some way, that perhaps some other patients who were equally desperate but didn't affect you in that way might not have elicited such a degree of commitment that you gave to this young woman.

John Davis: I think that's right. I think to my shame I would have to say that perhaps I would be guilty of failing some other patients where perhaps I was less guilty of failing this particular patient.

Windy Dryden: Did it have anything to do with the fact that she was a young woman?

John Davis: I daresay it did. She had a very strong bond with her own father. She was very attracted to older men and I daresay not having a daughter myself but only sons that I responded to her as a daughter, which complemented her response to me as a father. I could also be her knight in shining armour, Sir Galahad to the rescue.

Windy Dryden: So, in a way, because you seem to naturally take to this woman's situation for some of the more personal reasons that you have just mentioned . . . you seem on balance to have made up your mind to honour that degree of commitment that you felt towards her. Yet you said earlier that to your shame you might not have done so much for patients that you didn't feel so naturally drawn towards.

John Davis: Yes, perhaps I would put the boundary in a slightly different place with some other patients. I think one of the factors though, leaving aside the question of her being a young woman, and an attractive young woman at that, was the issue of trust. If a patient has great difficulty in placing any trust in another person, then when that patient does put trust in me it is that much harder for me not to honour that trust.

Windy Dryden: You seem to be saying that in situations like that, the negative consequences of breaking that person's trust would be that much greater.

John Davis: I think that's right. We are talking about patients who have very severe difficulties. Perhaps one needs to give less commitment to patients with less severe difficulties.

Windy Dryden: In circumstances like that I guess you feel almost like you are the only person in the world that the patient can trust and to break that trust might have in the long term negative consequences for the patient. He or she might find it impossible to trust other people if they can't trust you.

John Davis: Yes, without having fantasies of omnipotence I felt I was the only hope for this young woman. Speaking of hope there is perhaps one other kind of dilemma that I might raise in this case. There were times in our therapy when she felt that it really was not worth going on with her life. She was able to articulate this to me in a way which made the feeling perfectly understandable and there have been occasions with her when she left a session with me and I did not know whether or not she would be going away to kill herself. She would say to me that she could only tell me of that aspect of her experience because she trusted me not to try to stop her doing it. This was a dilemma for me. Should I allow her to go? How would I feel if indeed she were to kill herself? In all such instances I did allow her to go and took no steps to inform anybody or to prevent her from doing what she felt she needed to do. I think I always felt that because her bond with me was still alive that she wouldn't actually take that step and she never did take it, but I was never wholly confident about that. For me it always remained a dilemma.

Windy Dryden: You were gambling on the trust that she had developed in you?

John Davis: I was gambling on the trust, but I think I also felt that I really had no right to betray the trust and stand in her way.

Windy Dryden: How did that leave you feeling between the end of one of those sessions and the next scheduled session, not knowing whether she would turn up or whether she had killed herself?

John Davis: Well, as you can imagine, this kind of patient is very difficult to forget about. It is the kind of case that one carries around all the time. I don't think one wants too many cases of this kind on the boil, so to speak. I suppose I would simply have to say that working with a patient like this is demanding. It does use some of one's resources and takes them away from other people and other things that one might be involved in.

Windy Dryden: So you were preoccupied. You found yourself thinking about what might be happening. I am not quite sure what the quality of your feelings was on these occasions.

John Davis: It is difficult to describe. I think more than anything I would have to talk about it as having the sense of actually being with her, imagining myself inside her having whatever experience she might be having.

Windy Dryden: Did that mean that you experienced the same feelings of hoplessness too, at times?

John Davis: I think that's right. I think at times it felt as though the pain that she experienced was really too much. I felt that it was not right to ask somebody to simply endure pain of that kind and to hold out hopes that at some point in the future the world would be a less painful place to be in. Yet I knew very well from her experience that the fact that I could entertain hope for her was perhaps very important in that it enabled her to entertain hope for herself.

Windy Dryden: So it sounds as if because you could entertain that degree of hope for her that might have helped protect you from actually experiencing your own hopelessness about the situation.

John Davis: Well, the feelings of hopelessness were always tempered by that sense of bonding that existed between us. The hope lay in that bond.

Windy Dryden: So for patients like this young woman the bond between them and the therapist is crucial. That bond seemed to be the primary therapeutic factor in the whole of the therapy and any therapeutic techniques or methods that you employed with her definitely played a secondary role in this case.

John Davis: Yes, I think that is certainly true. Maintaining the bond of trust with this patient was of absolutely crucial importance, but then I think that maintaining the bond between therapist and patient is of crucial importance in any therapy. Of course it is especially important with more seriously disturbed patients.

DISCUSSION ISSUES

1. *Do you consider that John Davis is 'a therapist who has no idea where boundaries belong in his therapy'?*
2. *What general guidelines do you employ in drawing a boundary between your commitments to your clients and the commitments you have in your private life?*
3. *In what situations would you be prepared to cross this boundary to offer additional help to your clients?*
4. *Are there some clients who are likely to draw more commitment from you than you give to others? What is it about (a) you as a person and (b) your relationship with such clients that lead you to show this extra commitment?*
5. *What sacrifices (if any) are you not prepared to make in discharging your commitments as a psychotherapist?*

CHAPTER SIX

Where Are the Boundaries?

An interview with Brian Thorne

Brian Thorne is director of student counselling at the University of East Anglia, where he has been since 1974. He is also a partner in the Norwich Centre, an independent counselling and training unit committed to the person-centred approach -which was founded in 1980 and serves Norwich and the surrounding area. Since 1974 he has also been a co-director of the Facilitator Development Institute (British Centre) which has been active in introducing person-centred practice and theory to a large number of helping professionals through its annual summer workshops.

Brian has played a leading role in the development of student counselling throughout the tertiary sector of education and was chairman of the Association for Student Counselling from 1976 to 1980. Under his chairmanship the association established firm guidelines for the practice of student counselling and introduced its own imaginative and rigorous scheme of professional accreditation. Brian is the author of many articles on counselling and allied subjects and was co-author of Student Counselling in Practice *(Unibooks, 1973), which was to have a major influence on the establishment and development of counselling services during the 1970s. He was also active in the establishment of the British Association for Counselling, on whose accreditation committee he currently serves.*

Throughout his career Brian has been much concerned to draw on different areas of knowledge and experience in order to enrich his therapeutic practice. He believes that groups, communities and institutions have within them powerful resources for helping the development of individuals which often go untapped and unchannelled. As a committed Christian he has been particularly concerned to relate theological insights and institutional church life to the practice of therapy and his booklet entitled 'Intimacy'

49

(published by the Norwich Diocesan Board for Social Responisbility in 1981) is a powerful example of his attempt to move across traditional boundaries in the search for a more holistic approach both to therapy and to human living. It is this theme of moving across traditional boundaries that is discussed in the following interview.

Windy Dryden: Would you like to put the dilemma that you wish to discuss with me in your own words?

Brian Thorne: The dilemma concerns the question of the appropriateness of the therapeutic hour in terms of helping any given client. Increasingly I have come to feel that for some of the people that I see the idea of the traditional therapeutic hour, whether it be once or twice a week or— although this is something that I rarely do myself—three times a week, is not actually what is required. This constitutes a dilemma because it raises the question immediately: 'What is the alternative?' The more I focus on this particular issue the more I have come to realize that it actually strikes right to the roots of my. own therapeutic practice and my beliefs about therapy and human development. It certainly strikes right at the roots too of the whole question of boundaries, and what constitutes appropriate therapeutic boundaries.

Windy Dryden: What set of factors have led you to question the appropriateness of traditionally practised therapy?

Brian Thorne: There are a number of different factors. In some cases it is the growing feeling that for this particular client the experience of therapy is poviding perhaps the only kind of real antidote to a life situation and to a life history which have been, to a very large extent, destructive. I get the sense that in such situations the traditional help that I am providing is merely a drop in the ocean; something positive in the midst of a whole host of negative experiences both currently and in the past.

Windy Dryden: So it seems to you that this drop in the ocean is not enough?

Brian Thorne: It certainly seems that way to me, yes. As a therapist I often get the feeling that the client makes progress in the session but when he or she comes back it is clear that this progress has been completely put in jeopardy. So in such cases progress is two steps forward and one and three-quarter steps backwards. Although this may happen in many therapeutic situations, I am talking here about clients where the real handicap of negative past and present experience is very manifest.

Windy Dryden: You mentioned earlier that this state of affairs has led you to re-examine your therapeutic practice. Can you say a little more about that?

Brian Thorne: Well, in the person-centred tradition of therapy in which I work, it is often asked: 'If you profess that person-centred therapy is essentially about attitudes and a way of being, what distinguishes your behaviour in the therapeutic session from your behaviour outside of it?' So that is one aspect that is relevant to this issue. If I am able to be of use in some way to this client in the therapeutic hour and I maintain that the main therapeutic effect depends upon my way of being and the attitudes which I can actually convey to this person, does it not follow that what might be more beneficial for some clients would be to meet me outside of the context of the traditional therapy hour? That is one of the questions that is raised.

Windy Dryden: You seem to be saying that if the therapeutic hour is a drop in the ocean and thus not enough in terms of helping the client to cope with adverse and destructive elements in his life, then one of the ways of offering him exposure to a more productive interpersonal environment—namely yourself—could be to see him more frequently and outside the context of traditional therapy. Is that what you are saying?

Brian Thorne: Perhaps more frequently, but I am saying other things as well. I am thinking about ways of helping which are not normally perceived as therapy in any professional sense. Ways which may not necessarily involve my presence but which result from my intervention or cooperation. This may become clearer if I try to explain what I mean in some detail. Before doing that I have said that for some clients it is this 'drop in the ocean' phenomenon which prompts me to think there must be more that I can do to help them. However, I often have the experience too as I come towards the end of a session that a very productive rapport has been established between my client and myself, that some very productive work has been done and then suddenly the session ends. Now I know that it is possible to say: 'That may be well and good because the client goes away with a great deal of work to do. He goes out taking his unfinished business with him and that is splendid.' I am the first to admit that this may often be the case. There are other occasions though, when this situation is unsatisfactory and what the client requires is more space and more time at that point to continue the productive work with me that has been initiated. Of course, usually that cannot happen because the next client is waiting outside. So that is another point that I wanted to make.

To revert now to the issue of what other possibilities might there be for the client which would involve me, or might in some way involve my cooperation or intervention. I am thinking here of experiences which in many ways seem more closely related to and identified with the client's day-to-day existence. I don't just mean meeting the client say for a quarter of an hour in the coffee bar, although I wouldn't discredit that. I am thinking of situations where it might be possible for the client to actually offer something to me as the therapist. One of the things that has struck me is that very often clients *do* want to offer things to their therapists. In the past, I have often felt unhapppy, inhibited or suspicious of the client who, for example, wants to give me a Christmas present or wants to make some gesture of gratitude at the end of the university term. I have wondered about the appropriateness of accepting such gifts, although usually I have accepted them graciously enough. I am beginning to feel now that very often this may actually be something which is enormously important to clients in terms of the development of their own self-concept. They can begin to see themselves as persons who can offer and give. In the last year or two, for example, a number of my clients have invited me to tea, or lunch. These have been definite gestures to which I have responded and in some cases even gently incited. I have found that meeting the client in that kind of context has immensely enriched our relationship. What is of course much more important is that it has immensely enriched the confidence of the client.

So that is one thing. I take it further still. I have sometimes felt that what a client actually requires is not simply the therapeutic hour but the opportunity to spend *several* hours at one time with me; and not simply in therapy. In other words, I don't mean sitting for four hours doing unadulterated therapy, but rather setting aside a space of four hours which we are going to spend together. We might actually spend part of that time in a kind of conventional therapy session. We might then go for a walk in the country, have a cup of tea, and might end up doing some shopping together. It is almost, in a sense, irrelevant what we do. What is important is that we are actually spending time together because we have chosen to do that. There are still boundaries but different kinds of boundaries.

Windy Dryden: What kind of boundaries would you wish to set for yourself as you move into this new role?

Brian Thorne: This is where the dilemma comes in. I expect you have been thinking to yourself: 'He seems to have it all cut and dried.' Well he hasn't I assure you! I feel that this is all very tentative. I suspect at times that I am moving into a minefield and I get really very apprehensive about it. When you ask the question about boundaries it is there that I begin to wonder. I ask myself questions such as these: 'Am I really saying to some of my clients: I am not just willing for you to be my client, I am actually willing for you, in a significant way, to become part of my life? Which isn't necessarily to say I am willing for you to become one of my intimate friends, although it might mean that eventually. However, I am willing for you to occupy more space in my existence than simply the therapeutic hour.' If I am saying that then where, as you say, does the limit actually come? All I can say at the moment is that I am simply trying to be open to that question without getting too worried about it. Part of the reason why I have found myself exploring this issue in this way is that a lot of my work is done in a university where by definition I am going to see some of my clients around campus anyway. I also live in a surprisingly small city (Norwich) and there are therefore many occasions when almost inevitably I shall bump into some of my clients. What is also relevant is that I feel very much part of the community now, and I am likely to be here for some time to come. Some of my clients also fall into the same category. Instead of seeing this situation as potentially rather hazardous and a great drawback, as I certainly would have done some years ago, I am beginning to feel now that it might be nothing of the kind. There might indeed be something of a therapeutic advantage from living in this smallish community.

Windy Dryden: Coming back to the question of boundaries, do you think that there is a danger, perhaps, of offering more than you are willing to deliver in the final analysis?

Brian Thorne: That is perhaps the most pertinent question of all. I suppose one of my nightmares and certainly part of this dilemma is, in the end shall I constantly be having to say no because I have tentatively said yes too many times? I might be in the position of almost being eaten alive by far too many people, and then I would have to pull down the shutters. It is here that the presence of many other people who have some understanding of the nature of therapy and therapeutic work becomes very important. It doesn't have to be me who creates a new or alternative kind of environment for my clients. There are others, and they can become part of a much broader community—a much broader network. I think again that is where we are very lucky in being a small city, since as networks develop, such groups are possible.

Windy Dryden: It seems as if you have been able to expand your thinking in this area and apply it because you have been able to rely on such a network.

Brian Thorne: I think that's true. As I come to think about it, I know that one of my most important experiences as a young man before I became a professional counsellor myself was in a therapeutic community, as a temporary member of the staff. I became aware of what extraordinary progress is possible for some individuals when they are in a 24 hour a day therapeutic situation. What I am beginning to believe is that some of the advantages in that kind of situation can actually be replicated within normal life—within the residential life of a city and a university.

Windy Dryden: Right, you are not suggesting to a client that he or she go into a therapeutic community. Rather, you are suggesting that they enter into a community which is therapeutic?

Brian Thorne: Absolutely. What I might say to a client is this: 'You feel, perhaps quite rightly, that you are living in a pretty horrendous environment, humanly speaking. Your interpersonal environment seems to be full of destructive forces, and your past seems equally destructive. Well let's look now at the resources that are available to you. First let's look at the relationship you have got with me. Might it not have greater possibilities than this hour a week we spend together? Then let's look at this university, let's look at this city in which we find ourselves. Where might you go? Who might help you experience a far more positive and creative environment humanly speaking?' That is what I am trying to do.

Windy Dryden: So a client who has been exposed to destructive forces meets with you and you offer the appropriate therapeutic climate. You realize that this is not sufficient within the confines of a therapeutic hour, so you become more available to the client, and introduce him or her into a therapeutic network. I guess you need to be sure that this network is in fact going to offer the same sort of therapeutic conditions that you would offer in the therapy room and also outside.

Brian Thorne: Or at least approximate to it. I don't think one could ever ensure direct replication. However, I hope that the client may experience other groups, other people, other environments where some of those elements, which I hope I am offering to that client, will be present. My dilemma concerns how willing I am to offer myself outside the therapeutic hour, because I recognize that clearly there must be limits to that. If there weren't, I would soon be burned out and my own wife, family and close friends would see very little of me. To put it in very simple terms, suppose I see a client in the morning and I begin to feel increasingly, because I have been working with this client for some time, that it probably would be enormously helpful for this particular person to be able to meet with me in a slightly different context. Suppose I raised the idea: would he or she like to take a meal with me next week and the person said yes. Then in the afternoon I have another client and I begin to get exactly the same feelings. That's where the dilemma comes in. In a sense, who do I choose, when it seems so clear to me that there are many people who might be able to benefit from this? Now my hope is this. If the notion of the development of a therapeutic climate within various groupings, both within the city and within the university, begins to grow and become more of a reality, then in that situation I personally will often be very little more than some kind of stepping-stone or signpost.

Windy Dryden: But what if this development does not occur?

Brian Thorne: Exactly. If it doesn't am I, as you were suggesting before, setting off along a path which will eventually lead to the point where I am constantly having to say no, having promised to say yes? All I can say at the moment is that I am allowing this process to go on, and hoping that won't occur. I don't think I am being entirely foolhardy. But there are moments when I feel I probably am.

Windy Dryden: One of the aspects of psychoanalytic theory may be relevant here. When psychoanalytic therapists identify times when their clients feel rejected it would be safe in the knowledge that the client isn't being rejected by the therapist. They could then analyse the feelings of the client. You may very well be placing yourself in the situation where you are rejecting a client, or at least rejecting that client's offer to develop your relationship. However your clients may not be able to make that distinction. To whom does the client turn to cope with the pain?

Brian Thorne: My feeling about this is that if somebody makes an offer to me and I want to reject it, I would have to ask myself very carefully why I want to reject it. Is it because quite frankly I don't like this person, and I couldn't really entertain the notion of accepting an invitation to coffee or whatever it might be, or is it because that at the moment my diary is simply so full, that I couldn't conceivably fit another engagement in.

Windy Dryden: I meant a situation where you actually like the person, but that person wanted the relationship to develop in ways that you were not prepared to have it develop. I am thinking about the possible development of a sexual relationship. Let's further assume that you would choose to reject that and the client becomes very upset about this and turns away from you. If that happened in the therapeutic hour I guess at least you would have the comfort of the role of therapist around you.

Brian Thorne: Can I answer that provisionally because if I had all the answers this would not be a dilemma. I believe that I still actually do have the comfort of the role. What I am doing is extending, very considerably, the limits of the role. If a client very much wanted a sexual relationship with me, and that was something that I didn't want and I was quite clear about that and said so, this does not mean that I would necessarily, at that point, wish to reject that person within the relationship which we currently have. I think the difference here is that I am postulating a relationship between the therapist and client which extends much further into the day-to-day existence of the client, but without actually foregoing all the boundaries.

Windy Dryden: Right. What emerges from that is that I can understand that you would want to extend the boundaries of the role for the reasons that you have discussed. My point is this. Would the client be able to make sense of your expanded role?

Brian Thorne: I think that would depend almost entirely on the way in which my relationship with the client was being negotiated. I would certainly wish to ensure that as we explored the extension of the traditional therapeutic boundaries, some of the potential pitfalls are looked at in advance. Indeed, in the work that I have already done in this direction this has certainly happened. In other words, if it seems likely that an extension of the role outside the therapeutic hour is desirable and we explore the possibility of doing that, at the same time, we will begin to look at some of its implications, both before the event and after it. So, certainly, what I am saying is that I would expect both myself and my client to monitor very closely the effects that this extension of role was having on the two of us.

Windy Dryden: So you are describing a situation whereby the two of you both have an experience and closely monitor that experience?

Brian Thorne: Quite so. Let me give you a direct example from my current practice. At the moment I am seeing a person whom I have been in contact with now for three months and it is becoming increasingly clear to me that it would be extremely useful for us to have a longer period of time together, say three to four hours, principally because of how so many of our sessions seem to terminate. So often we both have the sense of having to cut off in mid-stream and are increasingly conscious of trying, unsuccessfully, to round off a session on the stairs or at the door of the counselling centre. She too is therefore beginning to feel that there might be great merit in the idea of more extended time together. We are just thinking about it. We are visualizing the possibility of that happening in a month or so's time. We are thinking about it—we are exploring it. If it gets to the point where we decide to do it, then certainly once having done it, we shall reflect together on what effects that experience has had on us.

Windy Dryden: OK. Let's take a situation where a colleague of yours was operating on the same principle. That person, in fact, was willing to explore the boundaries even further, and wished to become more intimate with their clients which would include sexual intimacy. Do you see any dangers in that?

Brian Thorne: I see enormous dangers. Yes. However, I wonder why you have put it as if it were a colleague.

Windy Dryden: Well, my perceptions may be wrong, but my sense is that you would say: 'I don't think I would go that far because I'm married and have a family.' Maybe I am wrong. Maybe you would go that far.

Brian Thorne: You are not wrong. You are right. I think you have actually hit again on a very important issue. It is something to do with the nature of one's own ethical framework or code of conduct to use an old-fashioned term—and how far I, at any given point in my life, sense a reasonable stability or security about that. At this particular time in my life I feel pretty secure about my ethical framework. Of course, I may be surprised tomorrow. But for the most part I think not. I certainly don't believe that I could be exploring this dilemma with you today, if it wasn't for the fact that I do experience that degree of stability and security about my own ethical and behavioural framework. Therefore to go back to your question about my hypothetical colleague, who might be wishing to push the boundaries much further than I would, then I think the question for me would be: how far has this colleague arrived at a point where he or she senses a reasonable level of stability and security about his or her own ethical and behavioural framework?

Windy Dryden: Are you saying that if your colleague would wish to extend the boundaries to that extent then you would question the stability of his standpoint underlying his or her decision?

Brian Thorne: I would probably raise questions about it, especially if it moves into the area of sexual relating.

Windy Dryden: Why?

Brian Thorne: Because I believe that it is within the area of sexuality probably above all that it is most difficult for any human being to know with a reasonable degree of certainty whether there is a real caring for and loving of the other, or whether there is in fact more of a sense of fulfilling a personal need. Is this colleague doing this for the benefit of the client, for the benefit of him- or herself, or for the benefit of both? These are crucial questions.

Windy Dryden: Of these three positions where do you think the therapist's position had better be?

Brian Thorne: For myself I believe that most of the time I am working for the benefit of the client. I believe that for some of the time I am working for the benefit of both of us. I suspect that if over the course of the next few years I explore and develop further some of the ideas I have been talking about with you today then I shall be involved in activity which more of the time is to the benefit of us both. I do not myself believe that it is ethically responsible for a therapist to behave in a way which is solely for his own benefit.

Windy Dryden: OK, but I can imagine a scenario where again your colleague (let's assume for the moment that it is a male colleague) has a genuine caring for his client and yet also finds her sexually attractive. She finds him attractive and also starts to care for him. That falls under the rubric of where the relationship has mutual benefits. Would you have any qualms about that?

Brian Thorne: I think I would still have qualms about it, yes. I would have qualms about it on another score. What would the effects of this behaviour have upon the community in which these two people live? Personally I don't believe that there is anything in the last analysis which is private behaviour. I believe that all our behaviour, however seemingly private, has repercussions on the community in which we live. Therefore, given the present situation in our culture and society as far as sexual relations are concerned, I would have qualms on that score. I am not though suggesting that there is anything in me that would completely rule that possibility out for my colleague. However, I personally rule it out for myself because I believe that although such behaviour might appear to be beneficial for me and my client it would actually have destructive repercussions within the community whether it be the close community of my own family and friends or the larger community.

Windy Dryden: I would like to return to what *you* are actually prepared to do. If I understand you correctly, with clients for whom the therapeutic hour is insufficient you are prepared to spend more time with them yourself and also to introduce them into a local community which you have confidence will be a therapeutic one.

Brian Thorne: Yes. Let me just repeat that spending more time with them may or may not be in what we may term a conventionally therapeutic way.

It is more likely to mean offering myself to them in a different way in a different kind of context as I have already outlined.

Windy Dryden: Let's assume that you work in an institution which may frown on that extension of a role.

Brian Thorne: OK, but I don't think I do work in an institution that frowns on it very much. But assuming that I do . . .

Windy Dryden: What implications would that have for you?

Brian Thorne: I think it might have considerable implications to the extent that I might not feel that I was able to explore this particular development of my work at all. The repercussions within the community might produce so many negative vibrations that any therapeutic benefit would then be put in jeopardy. So I am very sensitive to the community or society in which I live and work.

Windy Dryden: You are not then the kind of therapist who is prepared to stand out on a limb against the institution?

Brian Thorne: Not in that kind of way. My concern is to make institutions the kind of place where people are more likely to be able to develop as persons and if by my own behaviour I am actually producing more negative vibrations, more conflict, more animosity, then I suspect I shall not actually be improving the overall climate of that institution at all. I may well wish to stand up and shout in lots of different ways, through the conventional committee structure, through presentation of papers, or whatever. That is a different matter. However, what we are actually talking about here is acting in a way that would have a negative impact on the institution and I am not prepared to do that.

Windy Dryden: Yes. I can understand that. So given this scenario, we return full circle to the original dilemma where you only offer some of your clients help which is for them a positive drop in a negative ocean.

Brian Thorne: Yes. That's why I suppose as a counsellor who has spent a great deal of his time working in institutions, I see part of my task from the outset as working on the institution. It is because of that work and the impact that it has had that it is now possible for me to extend the boundaries in the ways that I have been describing. This institution is now much more prepared to accept that without getting itself into an agitated state about it. I believe, incidentally, that this is also true of the city in which I live.

Windy Dryden: Coming back to the world of reality then what you seem to be saying is this: I am more able to entertain this redefinition of my role because I have been to some extent successful in working on the institution and on the community at large to make it to some degree a more therapeutic one and also one which is now more receptive to my views.

Brian Thorne: I think that is a splendid summary, yes.

DISCUSSION ISSUES

1. *Do you consider that Brian Thorne is 'offering more than he can deliver' in traversing the traditional boundaries of psychotherapy?*
2. *Do you ever find working 'within the confines of the therapeutic hour' too constraining? How do you respond to this situation?*
3. *In what ways (if any) do you extend your work beyond the boundaries of traditionally practised psychotherapy? What factors guide you on these occasions? What do you hope to achieve in doing so? What are the risks of doing so? How do you determine that your actions are for the benefit of your client rather than for your own benefit?*
4. *Do you consider that there are any conditions where the development of sexual relationships between therapists and clients are justified on therapeutic grounds or do you consider this to be taboo? What reasons underlie your viewpoint?*
5. *What steps would you take if you discovered that one of your therapist colleagues was behaving with clients in ways that you considered unethical? What steps would you not take? Explain the reasons for your decisions?*
6. *If you work within an institution, to what extent do you allow this institution to influence your therapeutic decisions?*

CHAPTER SEVEN

In-vivo Intervention or Transference?

An interview with Marvin Goldfried

Marvin Goldfried is professor of psychology and psychiatry at the State University of New York at Stony Brook, New York. His duties include teaching graduate courses in therapy and assessment, primarily emphasizing the behavioural orientation, and supervising clinical psychology graduate students in psychotherapy within the university's 'Psychological Center'. He is presently engaged in research into therapeutic change processes.

Marvin's major achievements have been in the areas of behaviour therapy and behavioural assessment. He is the co-author (with Gerald Davison) of a widely used text entitled Clinical Behavior Therapy *(Holt, Rinehard & Winston, 1976). He was one of a small group of people responsible for the emergence of the role of cognitive variables in the practice of behaviour therapy and is one of the founding editors of* Cognitive Therapy and Research. *He has conducted research on therapeutic methods for the self-regulation of anxiety.*

One of Marvin's principal interests is the application of information-processing models, experimental cognitive psychology and social cognition to further understanding of the psychotherapy change process. Another of his major interests which complements that outlined is in the development of a comprehensive model of intervention that is based on the integration of the psychotherapies. In this regard he has already edited a major text, Converging Themes in Psychotherapy *(Springer, 1982), and is one of the founders of the Society for the Exploration of Psychotherapy Integration (SEPI). Together with Paul Wachtel, he co-edits the society's newsletter.*

It is this theme of psychotherapy 'integration' which provides the forum for Marvin's dilemma as discussed in the following interview.

Windy Dryden: OK, Marvin, would you like to put your dilemma into your own words.

Marvin Goldfried: The dilemma emerged within the context of a specific case and has re-emerged since that time with other clients that I've seen. As a result I can now frame the dilemma in broader terms. Let me start with the general case and then present the dilemma as it originally occurred, how it developed and how it influenced my thinking.

I have been approaching therapy from a cognitive-behavioural point of view, where, for the most part, the focus has been on the person's current life situation, rather than on his or her historical past. This leads to a review of the person's current life interactions and an emphasis on setting and evaluating homework assignments between sessions. The primary focus, then, is what goes on *between* the typical one-hour therapy session per week. At times however, an indication of the person's problem may emerge *within* the therapeutic interaction. The dilemma here is being able to recognize when this occurs and being able to decide when to focus on this in-session datum rather than on what goes on between sessions.

Windy Dryden: So it's a question of when to shift one's perspective from looking for maintaining factors of a person's problems which exist within the person's current life, i.e. a between-sessions focus, to considering that certain maintaining factors might be right there in the room with you, i.e. a within-session focus.

Marvin Goldfried: That's right. One of the constraints against making this shift, which perhaps we can discuss later, is that once we focus on what is going on within the session and within the therapist–client interaction, we are then making use of therapeutic orientation that is not typically part of the realm of cognitive-behaviour therapy, but is much more psychodynamic in orientation. This may very well account for the fact that many cognitive-behaviour therapists are limited in their ability to recognize this phenomenon when it occurs within the therapy session.

Windy Dryden: I wonder whether this in fact has to be the case. Just because cognitive-behavioural therapists choose to pay attention to material which is going on between therapist and patient, does their conceptualization necessarily have to be psychodynamic?

Marvin Goldfried: No it doesn't, but I must confess to experiencing a certain amount of initial self-consciousness when I shifted the focus to what was going on within the session itself, although, conceptually, I can very easily reconcile this with my more cognitive-behavioural orientation. Maybe this reconciliation might become clear after I have given a specific clinical example of it.

The first time this occurred—and I have become sensitized to it since then because I recognize that it occurs rather frequently—was with a 51 year-old male accountant with whom I was working. This man had a problem of depression, not only in his current life situation but had a long history of intermittent depression since being a teenager. In his current life situation he felt trapped, both in his relationship with his boss at work and in his relationship with his wife. He felt he was being controlled by others and was powerless to lead his own life. He had a great need to please others. The result of all this was a chronic sense of depression. Since he felt unable to *directly* control many aspects of his life situation, he would act in a passive-aggressive manner by 'fooling around' with other women or by not doing his job properly. This led to additional problems in his life, such as feeling guilty about not doing his job properly and his extramarital affairs.

My dilemma started to emerge when I presented him with a cognitive-behavioural conceptualization of his problems and a formulation of the treatment plan—both of which he initially accepted. He had been, I should add, in analytically oriented therapy for several years prior to this, but wanted a more structured and directive therapy, which was why he sought me out. Yet, once we identified the problem of unassertiveness as being at the core of many of his problems, and once I suggested that this was an area he needed to work on, therapy never got off the ground, despite his initial agreement. There was always something that would interfere. He would be forever bringing up other problems that would divert the course of the therapeutic focus. This was partly due to the fact that there were a lot of things going on in his life. It was also partly due to his obsessional style, in that it was hard for him to let go of things. His very deliberate and slow style meant that the sessions were sometimes very painful to get through. And part of it might have been a function of the fact that he was socialized to act as a patient in analytic therapy.

When I first tried to get some notion as to what the dilemma was, it was that he wanted help and wanted structure, but at the same time he didn't want these things. He would ask me questions such as, 'What shall I do?' or 'How can I handle situations differently?' and then when I would give a suggestion within a didactic, supervisory role, he would not always follow through on this. So there would be periods where he would start to assert himself more with people in his life, would back off, and other problems would crop up. He would then need to talk more about trying to understand why he was having some reactions, wanting to gain greater insight into his feelings. He thus wanted a more intrapsychic focus, rather than one which was more overt, behavioural and performance based. In thinking further about this kind of double bind that I was being placed in, i.e. with him asking for help from me, yet not really wanting it, it eventually became clear that the reason he didn't want help or suggestions from me, even though he asked for it, was that to him, accepting help meant that he could not help himself. Furthermore, he wanted to deal more with a lot of his past experience and with a lot of the subtleties of his emotional reactions. As I was trying to be more structured in helping him with corrective experiences that might advance his assertiveness and make him feel better, there was a kind of tension between us as to what the direction of therapy should be. It ultimately emerged that he was furious at me for controlling the therapy and not giving him what he wanted. His anger would take the form of his coming in and telling me of all the terrible things he experienced during the course of the week, rather than reporting any success experiences he had. When I tried to put the focus on his successes, he would initially comply; only later on did he realize that he was very, very, angry with me.

Windy Dryden: So it sounds as if you were getting a double message from him.

Marvin Goldfried: Yes. It took me a while before I realized what was underneath this double message. Even before I gained an understanding of what it was, I started to resolve this particular dilemma by becoming more passive within the session. I just let him take it wherever he wanted to.

Windy Dryden: You were stepping out of role.

Marvin Goldfried: Yes, I was stepping out of the role of cognitive-behaviour therapist who was teaching somebody coping skills. In the process of stepping out of role and really letting him take the lead, it became more apparent to both of us that he was reacting against me. He was acting in a similar passive-aggressive manner with me as he had with other people in life. For example he contacted an old girlfriend, after telling me that he was going to stop his extramarital affairs. He went back on his anti-depressant medication, after we both agreed that he no longer needed it. These were some of the indirect ways in which he expressed his anger towards me. After a while, the focus of the therapy shifted to what was going on between us.

Windy Dryden: I wonder to what extent the difficulty you experienced in stepping out of the role of a cognitive-behaviour therapist who was there to teach coping skills was accentuated by the fact that you have written on this topic and made a public statement on that score.[1] Namely that 'the core of successful therapy is the degree to which the therapist can teach the client coping skills'. Was this a factor at all?

Marvin Goldfried: Well, I don't think so, because I would still ascribe to that notion. And I still believe that the teaching of coping skills is what good therapy is all about. The problem here is how to define 'teaching'. Perhaps a better way to conceptualize this point is that the core of therapy is that the client learn coping skills. If we look at it that way then, as therapists, we became freer to explore different methods of facilitating the client's learning.

Windy Dryden: It still sounds as if you experienced some discomfort about stepping out of a more active and structured kind of role. Could you articulate this more?

Marvin Goldfried: I think what happened was that I became less active and more passive. It was important for me to be more of an observer of what was going on in the interaction, and less of a participant. As I became more of an observer, I was better able to see that what was going on in the interaction was very much the same kind of thing that was going on outside in his relationship with his boss and his wife, when they told him to do things. He resented that, did not want to comply but felt powerless. And because he felt that there was nothing he could do, he would get depressed, but also act out in passive-aggressive ways. As I became less directive, it became quite apparent to me that this was going on. Because I was a participant—too much of a participant, and not enough of an observer—I hadn't been aware that this was the issue.

Windy Dryden: I am still not sure what the basis of the difficulty or the discomfort was in moving from a participant role to an observer role.

Marvin Goldfried: Well, part of the difficulty was that it was harder for me to be an observer. It is much easier to see things outside of ourselves than it is to see ourselves in the context of an interaction. I think that part is self-evident, in much the same way that clients find it difficult to see their own contribution to some of their life dilemmas, and require an external observer in the form of a therapist to help provide them with that perspective. So I think that is the nature of the beast, indeed it is 'biological' in origin. Because our eyeballs are situated in our head, it is easier to see things outside of ourselves; were they retractable so that we could look back on ourselves, we could give ourselves a clearer perspective on ourselves.

Windy Dryden: Yes. I accept that. Although if you were a psychodynamically trained therapist, that is precisely what you would be trained to observe.

Marvin Goldfried: Yes. And that, no doubt, was a factor that made me feel uneasy about doing that. I am certainly well aware of the fact that this is the essence of a psychodynamic approach to therapy, and it was almost as if I was now abrogating my cognitive-behavioural allegiance and taking up a therapeutic stance that has been used by an alternative camp. I have been aware that this is an ongoing dilemma that I have experienced for a number of years in doing therapy. This may be getting off the track a bit, but let me just add a brief tangent here. Over the years when I have done demonstrations of therapy behind a one-way screen for students taking courses in behaviour therapy, I have noticed that I was very constrained in what I said and did. What I said and did while I was doing a demonstration was very different from what I would do if I wasn't conducting a demonstration. So it became apparent to me that I had been deviating from the constraints of a certain orientation over the years, and these experiences would bring home this awareness to me.

Windy Dryden: You became aware of the discrepancy of your public image from what you privately did in therapy.

Marvin Goldfried: Exactly. As I say, this has been going on for a number of years, and is in fact one of the things that got me interested in cognitive-behaviour therapy. It was apparent that cognitive factors played an important role in therapy, and that the more classic—if you can call it 'classic'—1960s behaviour therapy was not adequate to deal with what went on clinically. So, my whole professional career as a behaviour therapist has been characterized by many dilemmas all along the way.

Windy Dryden: Coming back to the case. Did that shift in emphasis help resolve the block that that seemed to have emerged?

Marvin Goldfried: Yes. As I said, what happened was that the client's resentment towards my structuring the sessions in ways that went counter to what he wanted started to come to the fore. A lot of the feelings that he had vis-à-vis other people were now expressed directly and openly to me; namely, that he felt powerless to control the session and direct its course, fearful of what I might do if he stated his opinion. He was enraged, but felt unable to express that anger. As we focussed on this over a period of several sessions, he ultimately did tell me how angry he was. This was a very powerful and dramatic experience for him, because nothing terrible happened. We got through that and re-established a therapeutic alliance with the two of us working jointly on his problems. This situation, rather than the one where it was him against me—where I was overpowering him as it were—together with the fact that he could express his anger and learn that nothing bad happened, opened up a whole dimension for him.

Windy Dryden: It sounds as if he was able to test out a pretty fundamental assumption with you that if he were to express his feeling then terrible things might happen, and yet he actually learnt to the contrary.

Going on from that, cognitive-behaviour therapists have not, in the main, addressed themselves very much to the notion of exploring the therapist–client interaction. I wonder to what extent you were operating under that notion with this man that what cognitive-behaviour therapists are supposed to do is to work on relationships between the client and the client's significant others rather than between the client and themselves.

Marvin Goldfried: My sense is that that is the typical procedure. At least I have not seen too much written about cognitive-behaviour therapy making use of the interaction. Now in books like *Clinical Behavior Therapy*, which Gerald Davison and I wrote in the mid 1970s[2], we recognized the importance of the therapist–client interaction as a potential sample of the client's relationships. *When* to deal with this relationship presents a different question. I had always operated on the assumption that when clients bring problems they experienced between sessions, we would work on that. Since that is closest to the criterion that we are working towards, that would seem better. In the case I've outlined, our relationship was interfering, so it had to be dealt with. Once we did deal with it, in fact, the client started to become much more assertive with other people and very willingly engaged in assertion training, focussing on people in his life situation apart from myself. Not only did we dispense with the issue of who controlled the course of therapy, but the experience of having risked stating his preferences to me in very forceful terms (he was aggressive and not assertive) and realizing that nothing terrible happened provided him with what Alexander and French (1946)[3] described as a 'corrective emotional experience'. He felt less depressed after having regained control over the direction of his therapy and he began to see the connection in a much more personal way between assertiveness and the absence of depression. Initially, when he accepted this formulation, he did so only superficially; he was still operating on the notion that he needed to gain insight prior to any change in behaviour. But here, he saw something from his own personal experience that convinced him that he could become less depressed in a particular situation when he had his say.

Windy Dryden: You mentioned earlier that this experience with this particular client sensitized you to the whole issue of the importance of dealing with the therapist–client relationship when appropriate. You mention this particular case in the sense that the interactional dynamics between you and the client interfered with treatment. Are you saying then that when there is, if you like, an obvious resistance, then that is the time for cognitive-behaviour therapists to address themselves to the therapist–client relationship? Or are you going further than that and saying that as a matter of course, cognitive-behaviour therapists would be wise to consider the here-and-now relationship as a microcosm in which the client's problems might occur?

Marvin Goldfried: I think the latter. The thing that sensitized me in this particular case was the fact that therapy was not proceeding. I think that there are other times when it would be wise to deal with the interaction between the therapist and client as a potential sample—a microcosm of the client's problem. I think it stands to reason that, under certain circumstances, and with certain individuals, the therapist will serve as a stimulus for the client's problems in much the same way as others in the person's life will serve as stimuli. To assume that there is no stimulus value for the therapist or the therapy interaction is to assume that therapy operates in a vacuum in a person's life, when in fact it is a very salient event. Consequently, I think that we should look at it much more seriously at times even when it does not seem to be interfering with the progress of therapy. If 'dealing with the transference' is an aversive conceptualization, perhaps we can think of it as 'in-vivo work'. We know that in-vivo interventions are much more powerful than imaginal or described ones. So if we can look at the person's actions right at the time—when they are being upset about something, or when they are being inhibited and cannot act in a given way or say something within the session itself—we have broadened our therapeutic focus. This, incidentally, is not at all inconsistent with a cognitive-behavioural orientation, even though another orientation might have 'gotten there first'.

Windy Dryden: Right, psychodynamic therapists got there first, in talking about the importance of exploring such 'here-and-now' data but the inferences they made about such data would be foreign to cognitive-behavioural therapists.

Marvin Goldfried: When you look at the notion of transference from a Sullivanian point of view, it is much closer to a cognitive-behavioural perspective.[4] He spoke in terms of parataxic distortions, namely that individuals have certain misconceptions of significant people that they developed early in life and carry with them to other significant people later in life. I don't think that this is a very high-level inference that involves 'repetition compulsion' or 'unresolved needs' or any other kinds of constructs of a motivational nature. It is really just descriptive.

Windy Dryden: Exactly. If I can move the tangent slightly, you are involved at the moment in developing the Society for the Exploration of Psychotherapy Integration—SEPI.[5] The way you have just spoken seems to me as if you are saying: 'Well look, I am still a cognitive-behavioural therapist, but I have expanded the range of data to which I am going to attend.' Would you say that was accurate?

Marvin Goldfried: Yes.

71

Windy Dryden: I wonder what range of experiences may actually lead you to change your self-description as a cognitive-behavioural therapist to, for want of a better word, an integrationist. I want to bring out the tensions that exist between adhering to a particular perspective as opposed to moving into the new area of psychotherapy integrationism.

Marvin Goldfried: That is an interesting question, and indeed another dilemma that I am often faced with when I work with clients. I ask myself, and also them, what range of experiences does one have to go through to change one's view of oneself? I think that it is a hard question for anyone to answer. It's hard for me to answer that about myself. I know that the existence of SEPI makes it easier for me to openly acknowledge that I am struggling with some of these dilemmas, mainly because I am in very good company. Having a reference group of other people whom I respect and who are similarly concerned with these issues makes it easier for me to openly acknowledge that I'm grappling with them as well.

There is another problem, though, in that there exists no other orientation with which I can identify. I have my own set of idiosyncratic notions, but it is really far from complete, and I would not dignify it by giving it a name or even by describing it in writing. It is still in its very early stages of formulation. It is so incomplete that I really can't identify myself as 'being that' or 'following that'.

Windy Dryden: Personally do you hope that the formation of SEPI, with its attempt to bring together 'fellow strugglers', will be a step towards the situation where people do not label themselves as belonging to particular schools of therapy?

Marvin Goldfried: I would hope so.

Windy Dryden: So we might actually see Marvin Goldfried at some point in the future stop describing himself as a cognitive-behaviour therapist, because you would share that aim?

Marvin Goldfried: Yes. I honestly cannot say that I am terribly optimistic that this might happen in my profesional lifetime.

Windy Dryden: I would like to think that this interview might perhaps hasten things on a little.

Marvin Goldfried: Well, maybe, but by its very definition, the integrative approach involves an integration of varying schools of thought in some sophisticated way—rather than the situation where a therapist says: 'I'll use a technique from orientation A and a technique from orientation B, etc.' We need to have a more integrative model of human functioning and human change, and I don't think any comprehensive one yet exists.

Windy Dryden: So you doubt whether integration will occur at a theoretical level?

Marvin Goldfried: Yes. I think for integration to occur, there needs to be a totally new theoretical structure about how people change that can account for the varying procedures that seem to work. The original behavioural model was inadequate, as is the contemporary cognitive-behavioural one. For example, it does not adequately deal with the emotions. An increasing number of cognitive-behavioural therapists are recognizing this, and a few of them are getting interested in the work done by experiential therapists. I find this development interesting and intriguing. I've had some fascinating experiences at an experiential-behavioural workshop recently, sponsored by the National Institute of Mental Health. It was organized by Barry Wolfe to bring together a group of behaviour therapists and a group of experiential therapists to dialogue on the processes of change and how such processes can be adequately investigated. As a result of this workshop, it became apparent to me that the affective components of a client's functioning are not adequately dealt with by cognitive-behavioural methods.

Windy Dryden: So you are hopeful that a series of these dialogues will actually bring together people from different schools so that the identification of a superordinate theory may actually emerge, that may actually help people to become integrationists?

Marvin Goldfried: Yes. I think, though, that it would be misleading to expect that a superordinate theory can be a combination of existing theories. I think that many people are put off by the interest in therapeutic integration because they believe that it is taking psychoanalytic theory, behaviour therapy and experiential orientations, and putting them into a blender and coming up with something that integrates it all. That is clearly not with it is all about. What we need is to reach some consensus about the common principles that operate across the therapies. Once we have identified a set of these principles that seem to be comprehensive, then perhaps inductively we can come up with some higher-level theoretical explanation that takes them into account. It is this middle level that we need to work at initially rather than at the highly abstract theoretical level or at the lower level of technique.

For example, if we look at the notion of helping clients achieve awareness, and look at subcategories under the general rubric of awareness, we can probably come up with principles that therapists could agree on as operating in the change process. If we take the instance where therapists help clients become aware that some of the unpleasant things in their lives—such as negative reactions from others—occur as the result of some behaviour pattern on their part, then I would speculate that most clinicians, regardless of orientation, would say that this is an important therapeutic task. Once we can come up with many of these kinds of principles, especially ones that have support from basic findings in psychology, I think that the enterprise of therapy is really going to advance beyond the point where it is now.

NOTES

1. Goldfried, M. R. (1980) Psychotherapy as coping skills training. In M. J. Mahoney (Ed), *Psychotherapy Process: Current Issues and Future Directions,* New York: Plenum.
2. Goldfried, M. R. and Davison, G. C. (1976) *Clinical Behavior Therapy,* New York: Holt Rinehart and Winston.
3. Alexander, F. and French, T. M. (1946) *Psychoanalytic Therapy: Principles and Application,* New York: Ronald Press.
4. See for example: Safran, J. D. (1984) Some implications of Sullivan's interpersonal theory for cognitive therapy. In M. A. Reda and M. J. Mahoney (Eds), *Cognitive Psychotherapies: Recent Developments in Theory, Research and Practice,* Cambridge, Mass: Ballinger.
5. For further information concerning the Society for the Exploration of Psychotherapy Integration contact: Dr M. R. Goldfried, Department of Psychology, State University of New York at Stony Brook, Stony Brook, New York 11794, USA.

DISCUSSION ISSUES

1. *Marvin Goldfried makes the important point that therapeutic allegiances may have constraining effects on therapeutic practice. What constraints have operated in your own work that are no longer present? How did you free yourself from such constraints? What issues did you struggle with in doing so?*
2. *How has the way you conduct therapy changed since you began your career as a psychotherapist? What accounted for the change(s)?*
3. *What labels do you employ when describing your approach to therapy? Have these labels changed over your career? If so, what accounted for the change(s)?*
4. *What elements of therapeutic practice do you currently not favour and why?*
5. *To what degree do you maintain a 'within-session' focus as opposed to a 'between-sessions' focus in your therapeutic practice? What determines your choice of focus in this respect?*
6. *What are your views on (a) therapeutic integration and (b) eclecticism in psychotherapy?*

CHAPTER EIGHT

On Leaving the Fold

An interview with Richard Wessler

Richard L. Wessler has been professor of psychology and chairman of the department at Pace University in Westchester, New York, since 1974. Concurrently, he practises at the Multimodal Therapy Institute and supervises at the Institute for Behavior Therapy, both in New York City. With Sheenah Hankin Wessler, he lectures and conducts workshops on cognitive-behaviour therapy in North America and Europe.

He received his doctoral degree in clinical psychology from Washington University, and held several academic and administrative posts prior to developing an interest in cognitive behaviour therapy. This interest grew from his realizing the limitation of the psychoanalytic and client-centred approaches to therapy in which he had been trained, and from his work in cognitive social psychology.

From 1973 until 1982, he was associated with Albert Ellis at the Institute for Rational-Emotive Therapy, first as a post-doctoral fellow and later as director of training and staff supervisor. He also served as editor of Rational Living, *the RET journal, during this period.*

He has jointly authored two books that have become basic texts in the training of rational-emotive therapists. He has instructed hundreds of psychological counsellors and therapists in RET and various forms of cognitive-behaviour therapy. Albert Ellis once called him 'the person who knows more about RET than anyone except myself'.

His current interests include the convergence and integration of psychotherapeutic approaches, to which he adds the usually missing spiritual aspects. His research interests are an extension of his clinical work, and emphasize naturalistic studies of therapy procedures and outcomes, and of how people have helped themselves through crises and emotional difficulties without professional interventions. His supervision experiences prompted an interest in how therapists make clients worse with thoughtless remarks, interpretations, and suggestions that disregard clients' moral principles and social values.

In 1982, Richard became dissatisfied with some of the more doctrinaire aspects of RET, especially Ellis's insistence on the primacy of must-statements in creating disturbance. His dissatisfaction with theory-bound therapy practices and therapists' routines that ignore diagnosis and assessment led him to decide to leave the 'fold' of RET and seek a more comprehensive therapy. In the following interview Richard discusses some of the dilemmas he experienced following that decision.

Windy Dryden: Would you state the dilemma that you wish to discuss with me in your own words.

Richard Wessler: It was the dilemma facing me, and in some ways still facing me, concerning my movement away from an identification as a rational-emotive therapist and recognizing privately and publicly that I have been doing something else for a good number of years. Also the dilemma concerning my attempts to put some label to what I have been doing, and letting other people know about this too.

Windy Dryden: At what point did you realize that you could no longer, in all honesty, describe yourself publicly and privately as a rational-emotive therapist?

Richard Wessler: I remember very clearly an incident which took place in the fall of 1981 when I was a visiting professor at the University of Leiden in Holland. I was teaching a graduate course in clinical psychology and I was making a comparison of the various explanations of anxiety offered by cognitive and other psychologists. I was discussing rational-emotive therapy and realized as I was speaking English very slowly that, first, I didn't really understand what the so-called connection was between the irrational beliefs and the resulting anxiety and, second, that if I did understand this connection I didn't believe it. In fact, I thought it was just preposterous. It was at that point that I started to recognize that I couldn't in good conscience continue to claim I was doing something that I was in fact not doing, i.e. practise rational-emotive therapy.

Windy Dryden: What did that decision lead to?

Richard Wessler: Well, nothing very dramatic; since I was in Europe and far away from New York there was nobody to confront me about what I was doing. However, I started having second thoughts about all the training I had done over a number of years. I realized that I had trained people in what I thought was rational-emotive therapy and had taught and advocated some of the basic theoretical principles of rational-emotive therapy and that these people were trying to do what I told them to do and I was in fact not doing that any more. These people believed the rational-emotive theory of pathology which I no longer believed, either. So, that was a kind of crisis of conscience I suppose.

Windy Dryden: Was this crisis of conscience accentuated by the fact that you, at that time, held a position as director of training at the Institute for RET in New York?

Richard Wessler: Not really, because I was on leave from that post. I was on leave from my university position as well as from the director of training post. So I really was not confronting any issues about it on a daily basis. However, the crisis was accentuated while I was teaching in Holland since they expected me to talk about rational-emotive therapy in a rather narrow way and I had never done that. I had always talked of rational-emotive therapy in a very broad sense. And, as it turned out, the sense was so broad that it was, in fact, meaningless. It wasn't until I came back to New York in the fall of 1982 and considered resuming my post as director of training that I realized that this just wasn't going to work out. I didn't think that it was going to work out even before I came back, but it only took me a few minutes of conversation with Albert Ellis for me to recognize that two different points of view could not be accommodated under the same roof.

Windy Dryden: And, what dilemma did that lead to?

Richard Wessler: Well, it was the dilemma of choosing between, in effect, recanting a heresy on the one hand and sticking by my guns and continuing to pursue my own course of thinking on the other. This wasn't an easy choice to make because it not only had theoretical ramifications but all sorts of serious personal consequences, and professional consequences as well. In effect, I was cutting myself off from the system that I had been centrally identified with for several years.

Windy Dryden: I see. Could you say a little bit more about those personal and professional consequences?

Richard Wessler: Well, on the personal front I encountered some financial impact since the institute and my identification with RET had furnished me with a significant part of my professional income. This was not only through direct payments from the institute for my services, but from other outside groups who would contact me. They couldn't afford Albert Ellis' fees but they could afford mine. Another personal consequence stemmed from the fact that many of my friends felt that they had to choose between loyalty to Albert Ellis and rational-emotive therapy and loyalty to me. The choices that some of these people made were very surprising. Some people with whom I thought I was very friendly now in fact shun me as if I am some kind of outcast, which I guess in a sense I am. On the professional front, I think anybody who breaks away from an established point of view (and RET is now part of the establishment) tends to be looked at suspiciously as though there is something wrong with him. A lot of people thought that I had simply had a personal fight with Al which was never the case. The criticisms that I have offered about what he has said and written weren't made out of personal spite or personal envy but rather made because I really and truly believe what I was saying and still do. Other people thought that there wasn't any difference in our respective positions and for a time only he and I and maybe two or three other people recognized there was in fact a very serious difference in our positions.

Windy Dryden: It sounds as if you had anticipated the financial losses, but did you anticipate the loss of personal friendship and the unfair criticism that you felt you received?

Richard Wessler: No, I hadn't. I hadn't anticipated that at all. In fact, as I said, I was surprised that some people chose to ignore me and I was also surprised that some people considered that I was simply trying to make trouble or trying to say something that would call attention to myself rather than saying something that I thought was really very important.

Windy Dryden: Looking back did you ever seriously consider saying something like: 'OK, I will lose money if I publicly disclose these differences.

Since I can't really afford to do that, or I choose not to do that, I will therefore fake it and keep quiet.'

Richard Wessler: No I didn't. I didn't think that faking it would ever be a viable option. I suppose I faked it in a sense when I fulfilled prior obligations to talk on and offer workshops on RET, since I tried to remain faithful to the point of view that I had been espousing and teaching in RET for some years. I would present the orthodox rational-emotive point of view and then suggest an alternative. At the end of the presentation I would confess that I preferred the alternative. But, no, faking seemed to be out of character for myself as I would like to be, as well as, I think, a rather poor practice for a psychotherapist.

Windy Dryden: Were there any other factors which have made this a difficult decision for you?

Richard Wessler: Yes, I think the most difficult part was no longer having a forum or a place to develop ideas. I relied very much upon weekly supervision, weekly contact with other rational-emotive therapists, to develop ideas, to keep the fund of ideas very fresh and I now miss this. I miss the supervision activity. I miss working with therapists, and training, very much. And I really feel cut off from everybody with whom I had been very close to professionally.

Windy Dryden: It sounds as if you have lost your place in a professional community.

Richard Wessler: Yes, that's right.

Windy Dryden: And what impact has that had on you?

Richard Wessler: I think it has retarded the development of my ideas. When I was given an opportunity to do supervision at another institute for a few weeks I found that my ideas began to flow again. I apparently need that kind of contact to keep my ideas flowing. I got it from listening to cases, working with therapists and facing live issues rather than from reading theoretical articles, research papers and the like.

Windy Dryden: You seem to be identifying two aspects of belonging to a professional community. On the positive side, belonging to such a community seemed to stimulate your creativity, and yet, on the other hand, from what you were saying earlier, belonging to a professional community was somehow a stunting experience for you. Is that right?

Richard Wessler: Yes. I think that is right. Belonging to the community, and not having an opportunity to step back from it and take a look at what I was doing, was stunting. I had certain obligations to fulfil—training obligations, a certain content to which I was committed as part of these obligations. These certainly were the negative aspects. So you are right, it worked both ways.

Windy Dryden: What thoughts do you have concerning the dilemma practitioners face in reconciling their theoretical orientations with the practical considerations of their daily work?

Richard Wessler: I think that practitioners do struggle to reconcile these two. I certainly did. I did from the very first time I conducted what I thought was a rational-emotive therapy session when I was a post-doctoral fellow in 1973. I struggled to reconcile what was supposed to be happening according to the school of thought with what was actually happening. Being less committed, at that time, to a school of thought, I paid more attention to what was actually happening and tried to help my client in a variety of ways. I was being eclectic partly out of ignorance and partly out of lack of commitment to a school of thought.

When I became more committed to a school of thought and became identified as one of its trainers, I tried increasingly to work with my clients from the frame of reference. However, I found myself becoming increasingly dissatisfied and began to make what many people thought were innovative interventions. I then tried to find some justification for these interventions which was consistent with the school of thought. Most of the time I was able to do this but not in every case. As a result I thought for a time that I could expand the rational-emotive school of thought and take Al Ellis' (1980)[1] definition of rational-emotive therapy as being synonymous with cognitive-behaviour therapy, literally, and include everything under this rather flexible umbrella.

Unfortunately, there is an inherent dishonesty in having one label stand for two quite different things. RET can't be at the same time both a narrow point of view about psychopathology and treatment and at the same time a synonym for cognitive-behaviour therapy. It can't both be general and distinctive. I justified my own activities as being general rather than distinctive but in the end such confusions and such muddles between the general and the distinctive just confused everybody: clients, therapists and trainers of therapists.

So as I was developing my practical ideas concerning how best to work with clients, I began to face the dilemma which arose from my actual therapy work becoming increasingly at variance with my position as a spokesman for RET. My conscience began to trouble me. Somebody who is a spokesman for a particular point of view I think ought to practise what he teaches, and I would apply this to Albert Ellis, myself, you, everybody. If we are going to teach other people a set of techniques or procedures or a point of view, then I think we are obliged to follow those ourselves.

I wrote to Bob Harper mentioning this point a year or so ago and he wrote back saying that he had known many of the big names in psychotherapy and none of them, as it seemed to him, appeared to do in their everyday practice what they advocated in public, and in educational forums. I think that this is shocking.

Maybe I am just a purist at heart, but I think that if we are going to advocate a position then we should be consistent with it. If we are going to teach others and tell them what to do we can't then say to ourselves privately: 'Of course, that won't work. I don't do it either.' We have to, I believe, say exactly what we do and not make claims to do things that we don't.

Windy Dryden: Do you have any speculations concerning why the big names in the field do not seem to do this?

Richard Wessler: They have a point of view which is associated with them. They are trying to promulgate their point of view, and at the same time they are trying to call attention to themselves because of their point of view. Big names get to be big names in part because they want people to know their names, not just because they have discovered something useful, good or important. I think what they do is, in a sense, become enamoured of their own ideas and what attention these bring them and aren't honest in telling people what they actually do. They aren't honest, I think, because if they were, they would lose their distinctiveness. People would say: 'Well you are just doing what everybody else is doing.' I think most of us in therapy are forced into a convergence of doing what most other people are doing. Where is the distinctiveness there? Why would anybody come to a workshop in which I get up and say I am doing what everybody else is doing?

Windy Dryden: What you are saying is then that novice therapists are being presented with a false picture.

Richard Wessler: Yes.

Windy Dryden: This seems to trouble you quite a lot.

Richard Wessler: It does. I have had the experience of novice therapists saying to me: 'Why doesn't this work? I am doing exactly what Albert Ellis did. Why isn't it working?' And what can I say, except to tell them that, based on private information—since I have worked with Ellis, have been in therapy groups he has conducted and because I have listened to dozens of tapes he has made with clients, both ones that have been sold through the institute and ones that never made it to the sale catalogue—that he doesn't do what he says he does all the time. In fact the RET that he demonstrates and people so eagerly try to duplicate when they become enthusiastic about RET is something he almost never does. And I think that is a very serious omission.

Windy Dryden: OK. But you seem to be saying that this is not just unique to Albert Ellis.

Richard Wessler: Bob Harper says that and I believe Bob, since he has known these people. I haven't known them.

Windy Dryden: It sounds from what you said earlier that you have always seemed to have worn the mantle of a rational-emotive therapist with difficulty. You have reflected on what you have been doing in therapy and tried to fit it into a rational-emotive framework.

Richard Wessler: I accepted the basic premise of rational-emotive therapy, about the effects of cognitions on behaviour and emotions. I still agree with that. I agree with many of the things Ellis (1962)[2] said in *Reason and Emotion in Psychotherapy* over twenty years ago. What I don't agree with is some of his later pronouncements giving primacy to the musts, the absolute imperatives, the shoulds and the oughts and so forth. I thought that the rules of science said you could revise theories as needed. And, the answer is that you can but you have to call them something else.

84

Windy Dryden: From the lessons that you have learned from this experience, what suggestions might you have for professional therapeutic communities and how they might actually benefit from your experiences in this regard? Also what are some of the obstacles that might actually prevent them from benefitting from these experiences?

Richard Wessler: First, I think it is important for all of us as individuals to have some support from a professional community. I think it is important in our personal lives to have support from personal communities, families and friends. I think we *need* them, which is very anti-RET thing to say. Professional communities are important to different people in varying degrees. Not everybody gets ideas like I do by listening to tapes of therapy sessions, talking to other therapists, listening to the points of view of other people, hearing the holes in those points of view and trying to plug the holes in some way. But I think that all of us are in a position not only to learn from each other but to have our work reviewed by each other, and I suspect we form different kinds of professional communities.

One such way would be in a work setting such as a hospital or clinic, another would be in a therapy institute where a particular point of view is being advocated. Now, at the Institute for Rational-Emotive Therapy I know that none of the supervisors and none of the therapists there practise rational-emotive therapy in a pure sense. I don't know why they don't acknowledge this. I don't know why they don't make a bigger issue out of it. In other words I don't know why they are still there. It seems to me that they haven't examined their position and I think a reason for that is the community itself because there is mutual reinforcement of each other's point of view—or what they think that point of view is. As a result of these assumptions and because it is a training institute where they are trying to convert others to that point of view, people there, and I guess this applies to other similar professional communities, don't take time to reflect on what they are actually doing, what they are actually thinking, and whether or not they are being as faithful as they can to a point of view.

I would like to see myself and other therapists become involved in less doctrinaire ways but this is almost a paradox. How can we be involved with each other in a less doctrinaire way and at the same time teach a point of view that we know very well? I don't know. I think the resolution to this paradox perhaps involves some compromise or perhaps just living with the strain of the thesis and the antithesis. Maybe there is no synthesis. Maybe there is only living with the discomfort.

Windy Dryden: Right, which is in a sense what this book is all about – living with the discomfort of actually wrestling with therapeutic dilemmas. One of the things that occurs to me as you talk is that you seem to imply that the therapists that you have been talking about are actually presenting selves as rather poor role models for clients.

Richard Wessler: Well, of course, we are entering the realm of values now when we address that issue. Is integrity an important thing for clients to absorb from therapists? If so then yes, many therapists are functioning as poor role models. If integrity is not an important thing for clients to absorb then, of course, it is irrelevant. I think it is a question of values at this point and I don't think there is any empirical evidence to sway it one way or the other.

Windy Dryden: But your position on this is that integrity is important?

Richard Wessler: I believe that integrity is important. And yes, I think in a sense that lesson became clear to me during this crisis. Integrity is important to me. And I have found that my own life is much more settled now that I have more parts of it integrated so that I don't have to fake either in my teaching or in my therapy—not that I really faked in my therapy. Also in my personal life, things are just a lot nicer for me personally. I wish it hadn't been at a price. I especially regret the alienation that has occurred between me and Ruth Wessler. Even though we had been divorced for some years we wrote a book about rational-emotive therapy (Wessler and Wessler, 1980[3]). I still like that book in a lot of ways; I said some things in there I still stand by, and yet Ruth chooses to follow a more orthodox line in RET.

Windy Dryden: What professional goals do you have for the future and what have you gained from this experience that would help you achieve these goals?

Richard Wessler: I hope to continue my personal development as a therapist. I think that it is very important for anyone who is going to teach others how to do therapy to have a good idea about how to do it themselves. They may not be brilliant executioners of it—that's all right. But I think that they should have personal first-hand experience, they should be able to work creatively and even though they may lack some interpersonal skills, some know-how and some other kinds of experiences, I think they ought to be able to appreciate the process of therapy and the people they are working with—not just from a theoretical standpoint but from a more comprehensive standpoint. If I were to do rational-emotive therapy according to the book, I would simply try to get people to chase their nutty ideas that prevented them from doing certain things and lead them to experience certain unwanted feelings. But when I work with clients I work much more comprehensively than that. I try to understand their lives in a much more holistic way, try to help them with some of the difficult dilemmas of life, and I am happy to say that Albert Ellis does this too, a lot of the time. I wish he would tell more people that he does this. So to get back to answering your question more directly: yes, I want to continue my development as a professional therapist. I hope that I have a point of view that other people want to learn about. I hope I have some experiences that other people want to learn from. I also hope that people continue to recognize that I have got a fair amount of know-how about therapy and that it is worth reading what I write and listening to what I say, for its thought-provoking value if nothing else.

In addition, and this is a special kind of mission, I want to correct some of the misconceptions that I was party to in those years of training people in rational-emotive therapy. Not that I think that these people are harming clients, but I know how personally discouraging it is to try to do something and find that it doesn't work. I would like to send a message to those therapists—namely, that they had better try to be more personally innovative. They had better try not to do it by the book, but be guided by more practical considerations.

Some people have asked me, am I starting a new school of therapy? The answer is no. I call what I do 'cognitive appraisal therapy',[4] largely because it seems unwise not to have a name for what you do. And I can't call it rational-emotive therapy anymore. I chose the label 'cognitive appraisal therapy' mainly to emphasize that, within a cognitive-behavioural framework, I especially try to tune into and help people understand their values, the appraisals that they make, the evaluations that are based on those values, to help them understand not only what these are but what kind of role these play in their lives, their behaviours, their emoting and so forth. I also sometimes use the phase 'integrated cognitive behaviour therapy' to show that I'm not only talking to people about their appraisals, or not only doing rational-emotive therapy without the musts and the 'shits'. Lately, I have joined the Multimodal Therapy Institute in New York, because Multimodal is a non-doctrinaire, integrated cognitive-behaviour therapy.

Windy Dryden: You seem now to be talking about your own struggle with distinctiveness. You seem to be saying: 'Well look. What I do in therapy is not the same as what RET therapists do, what cognitive or cognitive-behaviour therapists do. I do make a distinctive contribution, but I am not too sure what to call it, or in fact to call it by any name.'

Richard Wessler: Yes. I think that's right. I think you have analysed that very correctly. Partly of course it is ignorance about what other therapists are doing, and I suspect we are always in that situation. So much therapy is private, behind closed doors—and rightly so. But partly because I don't know of anybody else who is exactly, or even approximately, saying what I am saying: that I do an integrative form of cognitive-behaviour therapy, but that I give special emphasis, like rational-emotive therapists do, to the role of values and evaluations. I don't think I am just one of a kind, precious and unique, but I just don't know how many other people are doing the same thing.

Windy Dryden: And that's a function of being cut off?

Richard Wessler: Yes, exactly. I try to work in an eclectic fashion to be sure but it is not just eclecticism consisting of a little bit of this and a little bit of that. It is attempting to fit my procedures to my client's problems. It is an eclecticism that emphasizes the interrelatedness between cognition, behaviour and emotion, plus some other factors too that don't easily get absorbed in that triad—including the environment, and family, social relationships and the like. What I do is a lot like Lazarus' Multimodal Therapy to be sure, but even there I find that Lazarus doesn't seem to look at the interconnections between thoughts and feelings as much as I do. If he finds some irrational ideas he uses RET to get rid of them. If he finds some sensations that can be attacked through biofeedback and the like he does that. He doesn't emphasize the connections as much as I do.

Windy Dryden: It seems to me that in this interview you seem to be putting into practice what you were saying a little earlier about speaking your mind more even at the risk of staying isolated.

Richard Wessler: However, I am not totally isolated in that Sheenah Hankin, now Sheenah Hankin-Wessler, has been very supportive and perhaps comes closest of all people in the world to that other person who does what I do. So I would certainly want to modify any statements about isolation to take that into account. So I do have a community. Both of us would like a bigger community.

Windy Dryden: Right. I hope you find one.

NOTES

1. Ellis, A. (1980) Rational-emotive therapy and cognitive behavior therapy: Similarities and differences. *Cognitive Therapy and Research*, 4(4), 325–340.
2. Ellis, A. (1962) *Reason and Emotion in Psychotherapy*, Secaucus, NJ: Lyle Stuart.
3. Wessler, R. A. and Wessler, R. L. (1980) *The Principles and Practice of Rational-Emotive Therapy*, San Francisco: Jossey-Bass.
4. Wessler, R. L. and Hankin-Wessler, S. Cognitive appraisal therapy. In W. Dryden and W. L. Golden (Eds), *Cognitive-Behavioural Approaches to Psychotherapy*, London: Harper and Row (In press).

DISCUSSION ISSUES

1. *To which professional communities do you belong? What roles do such groups play in your professional and personal life?*
2. *Have you found that belonging to professional communities has had a stunting effect on the development of your therapeutic ideas and practice? If so, how did you respond to this situation?*
3. *Have you ever left the 'fold' of a specific therapeutic orientation? If so, what dilemmas did you experience on leaving the 'fold'? What did you gain and lose from breaking away?*
4. *How do you think you would cope with being professionally isolated?*
5. *Richard Wessler considers that prominent therapists often do not practise what they preach about psychotherapy. Do you think that he is correct? Do you practise what you preach in this respect? If not, why not?*

CHAPTER NINE

Who Am I to Teach Morals?

An interview with Peter Lomas

Peter Lomas is married, has three children, and lives and works in Cambridge. He trained in medicine at Manchester, became senior house surgeon to Sir Geoffrey Jefferson at the Manchester Royal Infirmary, and was a general practitioner for six years. He then trained at the Institute of Psychoanalysis, London. He has worked in a mental hospital, a child guidance clinic, a school for maladjusted adolescent boys and the Cassel Hospital, Richmond, where he studied post-partum breakdown and published a series of papers on the subject. This led to an interest in family therapy and in 1967 he edited The Predicament of the Family *(Hogarth).*

For the past twenty-five years Peter's main work has been as a psychotherapist in private practice. He is particularly interested in the nature of the psychotherapeutic relationship and has published two books on this subject: True and False Experience *(Allen Lane, 1973) and* The Case for a Personal Psychotherapy *(Oxford University Press, 1981). His criticisms of the current technical approach towards emotional problems have led him to seek an alternative to the traditional training institutions. At present he is involved in a teaching set-up in which students are encouraged to use their own initiative in finding the optimal means by which they can learn psychotherapy.*

Peter's aim is to understand the factors which stand in the way of an open and equal relationship between therapist and client and most of his writings focus on this question. He believes that professionals take for granted an unjustifiable superiority in conceiving what takes place between the two participants and explores some of these issues in the following interview.

Windy Dryden: OK, Peter, would you like to put the dilemma that you wish to talk to me about today in your own words?

Peter Lomas: Well, as I think about it at this moment, it is a very general dilemma concerning the question of where morality comes into psychotherapy. I am thinking particularly of the issue of how far one's own set of values actually influences what one is doing as a therapist. This matter is generally neglected in the literature. It seems to me that a therapist must have an aim for how he wants his patient to turn out to be. Although this question could quite easily be disposed of by saying that one wants the patient to be healthy instead of sick, this answer begs the question because one doesn't know what is the definition of health. Different people have different ideas about what constitutes health.

Windy Dryden: So you are saying then that the therapist's aims for the patient are more concrete than the vague notions of health.

Peter Lomas: Yes, I am. One can think in terms of health and sickness if there are fairly clear-cut aims that one might have in a therapeutic situation. If a patient comes along and says that he lies awake all night, then one would perhaps have the simple aim of helping him to sleep. However, in my experience with the people that come to me things are rarely as simple as that.

Windy Dryden: Presumably, the aims that you are talking about are influenced by the values of the therapist?

Peter Lomas: I think they are. I work in long-term therapy so I am not trying to achieve a quick cure of simple problems, because the people who come to me are usually those whose lives have gone badly astray, who have become lost and want to find their way in life. I have some idea in my mind of the kind of people I want them to turn out to be. I don't mean in detail, I don't mean that I may want someone to become prime minister or anything like that! However I think I have consciously or unconsciously the aim that I would want him to become the kind of person that I admire, the kind of person that I like, the kind of person that I might want to be with. I think that means that he would (if I can influence him) end up as having values about living which are rather similar to my own. To put it in general terms (which might seem rather pompous) I suppose I would like him to end up as a 'good' person in a moral sense, good according to standards that I, and perhaps many other people, would find acceptable, that many philosophers and religious teachers might regard as virtuous. Someone, for example, who believes in truth, who doesn't lie.

Windy Dryden: Now, in what way is this a dilemma for you? You are saying that your aim is fairly clear, you do have in mind what kind of person you would like your patient to be, and this is in part determined by your own values. Now, where in this topic is the dilemma for you?

Peter Lomas: Well, I think in two ways. First, because I don't set myself up publicly as a sort of preacher, a dispenser of morals, like a clergyman would who has a set of Christian morals. People don't come to me for that kind of thing. I feel a little as if I am a kind of priest in disguise — a priest in the very broadest of terms, not a Christian priest. It could be said that I am in the business of 'character building'. I don't subject my patients to cold showers or cross-country runs but I'm just as concerned to build their characters as the traditional boarding-school headmaster. Second, which is perhaps just a different way of putting it, I don't know that I have a right to impose my moral system of beliefs on somebody else. I wouldn't particularly like someone else to come and do that to me. I don't mind talking to people about morals and listening to people whom I respect talk about how to live, but I would not want to put myself in a vulnerable position where I might be influenced to adopt a set of beliefs which belong to them.

Windy Dryden: So, on the one hand you are saying that you would like your patient to turn out to be 'good' in the moral sense and yet on the other hand you don't want to be in a situation where you are imposing this value system on them?

Peter Lomas: Yes, that is right. That is where I feel the dilemma to be. I know I want to influence the person and I know I am going to try to do it. I can't help trying to do it. People come to therapy to be influenced in some kind of way and I can't just shut up and do nothing and leave them as they are. I suppose in certain areas it is not such a problem because if it is very broad then many people would perhaps agree with my view of things and the patient himself might actually hope to be changed in certain ways. Let us say that the person steals, then I don't, if it's a straightforward case, feel particularly uneasy about trying to influence him by whatever means, some of it by self-understanding, some of it by helping him to feel more secure so that he doesn't need to steal. I wouldn't feel much discomfort at having to argue my case for changing him into a person who no longer steals because I would imagine that most people would say that that is a good change; and he himself, particularly if he didn't find himself in court so often, might see it as a change for the better. However, I think there are many other situations which are not so clear-cut.

One such issue concerns the question of conformity versus rebellion, where there exist no laws, unless rebellion goes to an extent that laws are broken and people and property are damaged. I think that by nature I am a bit of a rebel, a bit of a non-conformist in some ways. People who come to see me sometimes talk about the question of whether they should revolt against a certain situation. I am thinking of a man I saw yesterday who had some dealings with a hospital as a patient. He questioned the doctor about his treatment, but was worried about making a nuisance of himself. He wondered whether he had a right to challenge the authorities or whether he should go along with what was being done. This seems to fall within the general framework of morals. It is concerned with how one should live, like the issue of the banning of trade unions at GCHQ at Cheltenham. One could imagine having a discussion about such issues and asking: 'What is the right moral attitude here? Should one conform as far as possible to the laws of the land and make life harmonious or should one challenge them and try to change them?'

Windy Dryden: Are you saying then that in the particular instance with your patient who is faced with a choice of whether or not to challenge the hospital system that because you tend to have values that favour challenge and rebellion that this might influence the way you discuss the topic with him, perhaps in the direction of encouraging him, albeit subtly, to take a challenging stance rather than a conformity stance?

Peter Lomas: Yes, I think that does happen and if it doesn't happen openly it happens, as you say, subtly. If I don't speak openly about my views, the patient will no doubt discern them by my responses, perhaps my non-verbal responses, my tone of voice, bits of approval and so on. I think my values will become evident. Whether I choose to make interpretations or not will be revealing. On the whole, like other analytically oriented therapists, I interpret things if I think that the patient's behaviour is abnormal or inappropriate in some fashion. Thus, for instance, if I thought that this man was challenging the doctor inappropriately, then I wouldn't come out with my own opinions directly, but I might make an interpretation. I might say: 'Well, isn't it an example of how you never came to terms with your father's authority, and you are still fighting him?' Whereas if I thought his behaviour was appropriate I don't think I would make that interpretation or any other.

Windy Dryden: So, what you seem to be saying then, is that the response that therapists make, like interpretations, are very much guided by their own explicit, or implicit, value systems. If that is so, since your values do affect your behaviour and since you do have in mind what you are trying to do with your patients, to what extent then do you publicly say: 'Look, this is the kind of person I am, these are the kind of beliefs and values that I have. These are the kind of beliefs and values that I think I would like my patients to have'?

Peter Lomas: I think that is a very relevant question, because one thing I believe very passionately about psychotherapy is that whatever the therapist does he must try not to confuse the patient. It seems to me that many people who come for therapy are confused; perhaps all of them are confused to some extent. They are not sure of their own perceptions. There are theories derived from work with families about how people have come to doubt their own perceptions because they have been placed in double-bind positions. I think that one of the ways in which a therapist can help a patient is to enable him to sort out these confusions. In order to do that I think he must make sure that he doesn't confuse the patient by, for instance, saying one thing and doing another. Or by pretending he doesn't have views—that he is quite neutral—when he really does. If that happens the patient will pick up cues which indicate that the therapist is incongruent and will become even more confused, especially if he is fearful of challenging the therapist.

Windy Dryden: So, you would not encourage the therapist to adopt a line of neutrality, because that would be confusing for the patient since under-neath this neutrality the therapist does have a set of values, and somehow by not making these explicit the patient will become confused—a situation which will presumably have a deleterious effect on his or her mental health. OK then, to what extent are you going to openly disclose your values?

Peter Lomas: Well here we come to one of the dilemmas, because to take it to an extreme, I would think it quite wrong for me to get up on a soapbox and start lecturing the patient about how people should live, telling him or her all about my beliefs. That would seem quite inappropriate because it would be imposing my values on them. And doing so when they are in a vulnerable state.

Windy Dryden: That's the 'imposing' model that you were talking about earlier and that's what you don't want to do?

Peter Lomas: I don't want to do it, so somehow, it seems to me, I have to find a way in which I am not shouting my views at patients or trying to indoctrinate them, but a way in which I am also not hiding my views to such an extent that I become confusing to them. I think many of the problems that one comes up against in therapy are rather similar to the kind of problems one comes up against as a parent with children. One has to find a middle way in which one doesn't try to brainwash people into accepting one's views, but also one would not try, as parents tend to do, to conceal things.

Windy Dryden: So, on the one hand, we have this 'confusion' model whereby the therapist has got values, and yet in adopting a neutral stance pretends that he doesn't have them. On the other hand, there is the 'imposing' model, the 'soapbox' model, where you stand up and lecture the patient about how he or she should live. Now, what you seem to advocate is some sort of middle ground. However I am not clear about the nature of that middle ground, I'm finding it elusive at the moment. I wonder if you could elucidate it?

Peter Lomas: I will try. I sympathize with your finding it elusive because I think it *is* elusive. It is something that one has to struggle with. I think it has a lot to do with establishing a kind of open dialogue with the person, in which as far as possible there is an equality. If a therapist is open he can discuss what is happening between him and the patient; how they are coming to the conclusions that they come to; why the patient might believe something; why the therapist, on the other hand, might disagree. If one is going to give the patient the optimum conditions for trusting his own perceptions then it is incumbent upon the therapist to be open. In other words, I think he should not only be open if challenged about how he feels people should live, but also admit his doubts about it, and explain to the best of his ability why he holds certain views. Then the two people could have a discussion about it.

Windy Dryden: Would this also include the notion that there were other ways of living one's life? For example, I can imagine with the patient that you referred to earlier you might say something like this: 'Well, look, in this situation because I value standing up and making a fuss I guess I might have done that. However, there are other ways. There is the way of X and there is the way of Y. Now I guess your goal is to actually find the course of action that fits in with your values, but I don't want to hide from you the fact that I value this course of action and yet I don't want to impose my views upon you.'

Peter Lomas: That's right. Yes I like the way you put that. It gives the patient a chance to make his own estimation of another person who he might respect and who is being open with him. However, he also needs to know in what ways the therapist might be prejudiced. He needs to be able to make his own critique of the therapist's position which would then perhaps help him to establish where he stands. As a result of this kind of approach (as you can perhaps guess) I do find myself having quite long and detailed discussions in therapy about such things as the morality of abortion. If a patient is thinking of having an abortion, the more traditional psychoanalytic approach would be not to discuss the merits and demerits of abortion but to interpret this in the context of the patient's personal history: to look for whatever in their own lives might have led them to fear bringing up a baby, with the result that they perhaps unconsciously are having the abortion not for the reasons they are giving but because there is some deeper reason that makes them fear holding a baby in their arms—or something like that. That seems to me the sort of interpretive method which I would criticize.

Windy Dryden: Which is based on the notion that the normative value is that the woman is naturally drawn to bringing up children?

Peter Lomas: That's right. I certainly wouldn't question an exploration of all the things that have gone into making the patient feel one way or another. But I feel there is an awful danger with that approach (as I think you are saying to me) of accepting a norm which the patient may need to be able to question.

Windy Dryden: Let's say as a result of this open discussion of values the patient chooses a way that for example is opposite to yours. So if you value rebelliousness he or she might choose the conforming way; if you value truth he or she might choose the deceptive way. Is that a dilemma for you?

Peter Lomas: Yes.

Windy Dryden: In what way?

Peter Lomas: It is a dilemma because I don't know how far I should let the patient go his own way—a way which I don't approve of. I don't know how far I should try to stop him. In a way it is the question of how much one stands back, feeling that the person's freedom is very important even if he is going to do something that appears to you self-destructive.

Windy Dryden: Which is a value in itself?

Peter Lomas: Yes. A freedom to live one's own life however one does it. It is a value. So I am torn between letting that happen and saying nothing or pointing out ways in which I think they might be misguided, ways which might lead them into trouble. These are very similar dilemmas to those one has in ordinary life with one's family and friends; it is just that I think in psychotherapy they tend to be obscured by theory. In day-to-day psychotherapy such matters as whether one should marry somebody or not are being discussed as they would with one's family and friends.

Windy Dryden: I wonder if one of the theories which tends to obscure this problem in psychotherapy is the theory that states that the preferred role of the therapist should be that of a facilitator. This theory states that the goal of the therapist is not to impose or even necessarily bring out one's own value systems but to help the client find their own way no matter what way that might turn out to be. Perhaps most of the time the client may find a way which society in general would call 'good' and moral but at times the client would go off in a self-destructive way and if that happens so be it. It is not necessarily the therapist's task to say: 'Hey wait a minute but that's the wrong way.' Is that one of the theories that might obscure this issue, would you say?

Peter Lomas: I think it does. I think it obscures the issue because it implies that one can be a neutral facilitator. First, I don't believe one can be neutral and, second, I believe even if one takes a neutral stand it could at times be immoral to sit back and let someone do something very destructive. The ultimate example would be suicide. If one really thought a patient would commit suicide and was going to do so for stupid reasons, sick reasons, it would seem to me that I would want to do something or say something to stop him. I might even take drastic action.

Windy Dryden: What implications does what you are talking about have on the way therapists actually establish a therapeutic enterprise with their patients?

Peter Lomas: I think quite a lot, because the way the therapist behaves and the expectations he has of the patient show to quite a degree, I think, his moral stance in life, and in society. Whether for instance he believes that people are equal; whether he believes in hierarchies; what his attitude is to professionalism; what his attitude is to intimacy; to what extent he feels people should be open and close with each other, or not; what he believes about money. The way he dresses is as revealing as is the way he speaks to the client. Does he for example believe in gentleness or roughness? Is he a permissive kind of person who is going to give a lot of space to the patient, or is he someone who will go in for a lot of confrontation and challenge? These issues might have something to do with his theoretical beliefs and technique, it might be something to do with his personality—the way he is made—but it also seems to be something to do with the moral stance he takes about how people should behave with each other.

Windy Dryden: If you set up a psychotherapeutic enterprise, where you are going to make explicit these things, you may very well lose a number of clients, who for example don't think it is your job to actually disclose your beliefs, or want you to act in a different way, or don't value at the beginning the kind of things that you value. Therefore you cannot establish a therapeutic alliance with them.

Peter Lomas: Well, I find that rather rare. I find that when people come to me they don't usually break off, and I suspect that part of that has to do with selection.

Windy Dryden: I was just going to mention that. Your referral network might be helpful in this respect in that they might say: 'We'll send this person to Peter, he or she is the sort of person who we think is going to get on with Peter, is going to share some of his beliefs.'

Peter Lomas: I think that is true. This wouldn't happen if I was working in the Health Service; I have worked for the Health Service in the past so I've some experience of that kind. It would be less likely to happen if I were working in London rather than in a relatively small city where people can get to know me and my beliefs. And it is likely to happen because I write. Quite a number of my clients come to me because they have either read what I have written or because they have been recommended to me by a friend. So I think there is a certain amount of selection in that. It would be rather nice for me to believe that I was such a great therapist that people don't break off. That could have its hazards couldn't it? It could be that I collude in some way to keep them, but yes, I think selection plays a big part in what you mention.

Windy Dryden: So therapists who work more anonymously had better face the fact then that if they are going to openly disclose values, and conduct therapy according to these values, they may not be able to establish a therapeutic alliance with clients who at the very outset are going to share a different morality, a different value system so that coming together may not be viable?

Peter Lomas: It may be a problem. I haven't thought of it as much of a problem because it is not as though a therapist working as I do gets particularly known for, say, his political beliefs. If I were a very strong Marxist, for instance, then that could lead me into trouble, but even if I were I don't think I would announce it.

Windy Dryden: However, if you were a Marxist and a client was talking about adding yet another factory to his empire that might cause you a dilemma.

Peter Lomas: Yes, I think it would, and I think I would have to be tactful. That might sound a rather unscientific, messy and uncourageous way of doing it, but I think that particularly at the early stages with a client if one confronted him very quickly with diametrically opposed views then one might lose him or it might be so upsetting that he would shut up; and that wouldn't be therapeutic. However, the sooner I could get to telling them where I stood the better.

Windy Dryden: So let me see if I can sum up what you seem to be talking about today. As a therapist you neither want to impose values on your clients, nor do you want to remain neutral. You want to actually let patients know where you stand on things, you want to show that there are alternatives, and that when they take those alternatives that is a dilemma for you because it confronts you with the notion that patients may proceed in ways that you from your value system deem to be self-destructive, and in this circumstance you may very well try to stop them doing this. Does that seem to be the way that you have actually solved this dilemma for yourself?

Peter Lomas: Yes, there are certainly instances where I would not disclose.

Windy Dryden: What might some of these instances be?

Peter Lomas: Well I suppose they would be instances in which I would feel perhaps insecure in my own view and so I would let the thing go for better or for worse. It also occurs to me that I would hold back my own view sometimes if I thought it was going to be particularly painful, traumatically painful, to another person. If somebody had done something which I thought was a heinous crime I might play that down because I wouldn't want at that moment to increase the guilt he already feels. I would hope later on, when he was in better shape, that we would discuss it more openly and both admit that what had been done was terrible.

Windy Dryden: I guess from what you were saying earlier, there is always a risk in so doing that the patient is going to be confused, because on the one hand you are not giving a view and yet they may sense that view.

Peter Lomas: Yes I would feel very uneasy doing that and I do it to the very minimum. I'm only saying that sometimes I do do it.

Windy Dryden: So there are pragmatic grounds which may intervene and stop you from saying: 'Well, this is my moral principle.'

Peter Lomas: That's right. If there's one thing that guides me in this it's the thought that I must use common sense in therapy just as much as in ordinary living.

DISCUSSION ISSUES

1. *To what extent do you consider that therapists can be neutral facilitators of their clients' personal development?*
2. *To what degree do your own personal values influence your therapeutic practice? Which values in particular are most influential in this respect? What dilemmas (if any) does this pose for you? How have you attempted to resolve these dilemmas?*
3. *What is your image of the 'good' person, in the moral sense?*
4. *To what extent do you hope that your clients will turn out to be 'good' persons at the end of therapy? How do you respond to clients who seem to be changing in ways you disapprove of?*
5. *To what degree do you openly disclose your values to clients? What guides you in this this respect?*

CHAPTER TEN

Splitting and Integration in Marital Therapy

An interview with Paul Brown

Paul Brown is both a clinical and an occupational psychologist. This creates a division in the way he uses his time but not in his essential interests, which are to do with the individual's capacity to realize potential.

His work beyond the confines of the NHS started twelve years ago, when he resigned his NHS and university appointments to pursue a personal experiment in how a clinical psychologist might survive in a freelance or self-employed manner. That experiment has included periods of research for the National Marriage Guidance Council, being a managing director of a career counselling organization, directing the psychological services of the same company, and pursuing the politics of professional associations, as well as private clinical practice throughout the whole period. He was the founding chairman of the Association of Sexual and Marital Therapists; proposed the formation of the Counselling Section of the British Psychological Society; and has just completed a period as chairman of the Association of Clinical Psychologists in Private Practice. He is co-editor of a new journal entitled Sexual and Marital Therapy, *and is the review editor for the* British Journal of Guidance and Counselling. *His own publications include co-authoring* Treat Yourself to Sex *(Penguin, 1979).*

Organizationally he now works in process consultancy in career reassessment and development, and in understanding the nature of the relationship of subordinates to their superiors in organizations. Clinically he works especially in sex and marital therapy. His professionally independent position and willingness to explore the boundaries of attachment to and separation from organizations is reflected in the following interview.

Windy Dryden: OK, Paul, would you like to put the dilemma you wish to discuss with me in your own words?

Paul Brown: It occurs in this kind of situation. A single individual or a couple will come to see me seeking marital therapy and either in the first session or in a subsequent session ask directly for my opinion as to whether or not their marriage is at an end. A related dilemma appears when a couple come into therapy in a high-conflict situation after typically having already seen a number of therapists. In this situation everything about the relationship screams out to me that there is no productive future in this marriage. One can see how it might be maintained at a psychopathological level but not at a productive level. The dilemma then is whether or not in the context of that encounter I should say to the couple something along these lines: 'It seems so obvious to me that this marriage is at its end that I wonder whether we shouldn't take that as our starting point.'

Windy Dryden: Does the first situation you mentioned occur at the beginning of a therapeutic encounter?

Paul Brown: The first situation can be at the beginning or can be in the process of therapy. The distinctive feature of this situation is that the individual or the couple directly asks for my opinion concerning the viability of the marriage.

Windy Dryden: In the second situation the person or couple doesn't necessarily ask you directly for your opinion but it is clear from your perspective that the relationship from a productive point of view is just not working out. OK, let's take these one at a time. What is your dilemma in the situation where you are asked directly for your opinion?

Paul Brown: Well, the first situation relates to the nature of psychological understanding as a predictive science. If we take some of the physical sciences like bridge building or airplane construction, where major accidents have happened in the past and are likely to happen again, a great deal of effort is put into determining why such effects have occurred. Information thus gained is then built into future safety regulations and standards and so on. However this approach rarely occurs in relation to the psychological sciences. And yet, when one thinks of the disasters that occur for example in many marriages one wonders why we don't approach such matters in this way.

Now when an individual—and I think this situation more typically happens when a single individual comes into therapy—asks, 'Do you really think my marriage is at an end?', a counselling approach would normally involve reflecting that question back to the person. The question is taken as a statement that the person wishes to hear reflected so that he or she can explore it further. Yet it also seems to me that there are times when it is unkind and anti-therapeutic for me not to reveal my own view of the situation, if that view is well founded. In my own therapeutic practice I am increasingly conscious that one can have thoroughly well-founded views that lead to quite clear conclusions and it is dishonest not to disclose these if asked. It is similar to the situation where a patient says to a physician: 'Tell me if I have got cancer so that I can grapple with it.' If the physician dodges the question he or she may be depriving the individual of an opportunity to cope constructively with the illness. The question about the death of a relationship presents a conflict for me as a practising clinician because of the split within me between the scientist/clinician part of me—my original training was in this mode—and the psychotherapist part which reflects more my style of current practice.

Windy Dryden: So there are two issues here. When somebody asks you directly for your opinion about the viability of a relationship your dilemma is this: to what extent can I answer this question as a scientist drawing on a sound body of scientific knowledge of relationships, and to what extent am I going to respond to this question from my perspective as a psychotherapist whose major task is to help the person explore such concerns and come to a decision from their own perspective?

Paul Brown: Yes, I think that's right. Yes. Of course it is sometimes the case that one can see that the person has asked the question out of feelings of confusion, doubt, anxiety or fear. In a way that is easier to deal with, because it is clear that the question is appropriate in its context. What is more difficult is when the person says straight out, 'Is my marriage at an end?', and the dilemma of course only arises if one has formed a view. I am not at that point comfortable with staying simply within the counselling style when in fact I do have a view about it.

Windy Dryden: Could you perhaps give an example that might illustrate what you are saying?

Paul Brown: Yes. A woman of 43 came along nine months ago saying that she wanted to be more sexual in her marriage. Throughout the history of her marriage she had never enjoyed sex, had permitted sexual encounters only about once a month and knew that it had been a bone of contention in the marriage. Otherwise it was a happy marriage. The husband, a retailer, was productively engaged in work. They had a good style of life and a large circle of friends. However, because the children were now approaching their early twenties, she felt that the question of their unsatisfactory sexual relationship was really coming more to the fore, and that now was the time when she ought to begin to deal with it. It transpired in the course of the initial sessions that in fact she felt that her husband had rather withdrawn his affection from her over the previous two years and it was this that had instigated the search for help.

Therapy was beginning to involve a broadly based exploration of her wider concerns about her marriage, rather than being focused upon sexual function, though it is quite interesting as an aside to note that hormonal investigations showed that she had hyperprolactinaemia, which is bad news from the point of her own spontaneous arousal. Then her husband disappeared for three weeks, and it eventually transpired that he had gone off to France to think things over. She had suspected that he had been having an affair but couldn't find any evidence for her suspicions and he had denied it. In due course I invited the husband into therapy in order to try and understand his experience of the relationship. He came willingly and we discussed the issue of whether or not he was having a relationship with anyone else. There was no evidence that I could deduce that this was the case. Yet the marriage seemed to be very blocked. The husband was not giving anything, and the woman felt very isolated and cut off. Most of her friends were saying to her: 'Well it is time you got out of this marriage.' At that point she asked me directly, 'Do you think our marriage is at an end?', though not in his presence.

Windy Dryden: Did you have a view about that?

Paul Brown: Well it happened in this particular instance that I did have a view that their marriage was not at an end and, in fact, said so. It transpired about ten months later that indeed the husband had had a major affair for the previous two years, which he had managed to keep completely secret. We have now worked through that and they have in fact decided to re-establish their marriage. There was good reason for that since, despite their problems, they seemed to have a lot of warmth and a lot of support for one another. There was a lot of caring. There wasn't much sex, but there was a lot of caring and support. On that basis I suggested that their marriage in fact was very viable.

Windy Dryden: Did you find it difficult to say that?

Paul Brown: Not at all. However, subsequently I wondered what I would have said at that juncture if I had formed the view that the marriage was in fact at an end.

Windy Dryden: Now, at that point, presumably from what you were saying before, your dilemma would actually have come to the fore. I sense that you weren't struggling that much before saying to her: 'No I think there is hope for your marriage.' What would stop you from saying: 'From looking at the various areas in your marriage it doesn't seem to me that very many of your desires are being met and it seems to me that your marriage is at an end'? What would you be struggling with there?

Paul Brown: That is a good question. I suppose as a therapist I really get quite involved in what is happening to the people I am working with, and invest quite a lot of hope in their well-being. It seems to me that the break-up of a marriage is a painful, difficult and bleak affair, like an amputation that leaves the pain of a phantom limb particularly if there are children around, with all the separating that goes on. It is a painful event for me as well as for the patient although it happens often enough for me to know what that journey is like. So I think in part, though I haven't actually ver-bilized it in these terms before, that my hesitation about making an authoritative statement which encourages the split to happen revolves around the difficulty of coping with the ensuing pain. Also, because these things are rarely absolute, there might be a 20 per cent chance that the relationship could improve. If there is a good therapeutic relationship and a high level of trust, if I did give a definite view that was strongly weighted on balance towards saying that the marriage was at an end, my sense is that the person would take that on board and use it as a very crucial piece of infor-mation that might influence him or her quite profoundly. As I don't personally like using paradoxical effects I would never say something like that just in order to try and produce a therapeutic effect.

Windy Dryden: Right, so there are two elements here. First if you were to say, 'I think from what you are saying it seems that your marriage is at an end,' then you and the patient will have to face the hopelessness and despair that a break-up of a marriage would bring. Second, you may actually hasten that split by making that kind of authoritative statement. And yet you do not hesitate to hasten a reconciliation by making an authoritative statement to the effect that: 'I think there is hope for your marriage.'

Paul Brown: That's again an interesting observation. I am reminded of the fact that in the particular case that I have been describing, the husband would have been quite pleased I think to hear me say, 'I think your marriage is at an end,' because it would have given him the permission he was seeking, i.e. to go off with his mistress—a dilemma which he subsequently struggled with before deciding not to go. At that point had I said something to doubt the viability of the marriage then I think he would have gone and his wife would have been bereft. They certainly wouldn't have got to the stage of rebuilding their relationship. Although in principle one likes to think of oneself as neutral in the therapeutic encounter, in practice I don't think I have ever been productively involved in therapy where I have actually felt neutral. Consequently, one is simultaneously in the position of the scientist-observer who tries to be objective and the engaged therapist whose feeling processes are inevitably highly tuned-in, so one is trying to integrate the observational and the involved sides of oneself. It is a bit like the scientist who is doctoring his experiments or the area of experimenter expectancy. Sometimes it seems to me that therapy has got that element in it. Because of one's involvement in the situation one may well be at risk of producing the results that one would like to see without maintaining objectivity. There is a point at which understanding—the scientist's role—has to move into intervention—the committed therapist's role.

Windy Dryden: So since you don't believe you are being neutral in therapy, you would like to doctor the data in favour of making statements that may actually perpetuate the life of a relationship rather than statements that might actually initiate its death?

Paul Brown: I hadn't thought of that before. I think I do move into most therapy encounters conveying the sense of optimism that human beings can develop, change, grow, come together and discover the positive aspects of each other.

Windy Dryden: OK, let's deal with the situation where even your optimism for a particular case runs out and where you are quite convinced in your mind that a particular relationship has reached an end.

Paul Brown: Well, let me give you an example of that. A couple again in their late forties were referred to me by a marriage counsellor who had been seeing them somewhat unwillingly for about eighteen months. The counsellor had been seeing them because a physician who was both a friend of the counsellor and the couple had suggested to both parties that it would be a good idea. The counsellor actually hadn't wanted to see them but felt obliged to the physician and saw the couple fortnightly for eighteen months. He was an accountant, she a lawyer. He had spent twenty-five years of their marriage, until four years prior to coming to see me, very actively involved in local politics for four nights a week. She had been pretty much left alone to raise a family and as the children got older she had gone back into law practice and became quite well known in local circles as a feminist lawyer of the angry variety. If a woman wants to screw her husband for everything that she can get by way of settlement it is well known that this lawyer will fight tooth and nail on the woman's behalf. This couple came to see me at the counsellor's request. The woman in the couple had also by that time been in once weekly analytic psychotherapy for about a year and the husband had been in analytic therapy for a couple of months and they both came with the knowledge of their separate therapists. At the time when the man had ceased his involvement in local politics, he had also been squeezed out of his partnership in his firm of accountants and another partnership that he had subsequently joined was really not working out for him and he was feeling very lost professionally.

I have never sat through a therapy hour with two such hostile, bitter, fighting people. Their marriage had reached its crisis because the husband had discovered that his wife had been having an affair for about three years during the time that he had ostensibly given up politics to devote more time to home. He had recently wrung a promise out of her to give up this relationship which as far as we could tell she had done, albeit unwillingly. However that relationship was still an option for her.

About half an hour into this first session every test that one could apply about what a working productive marriage might be revealed that this relationship was sadly failing. What I said was: 'It is really quite important at this stage of our meeting for me to offer you a view which is that so far as I can tell your marriage is as dead a marriage as I have ever seen. There is no future in it and perhaps the real task is for you to discover together how you can separate in a way that leaves some residual regard for each other.' That is not a statement that I often make. But it was very productive in one sense in that it revealed that each of them was feeling very frightened. They were both terrified as to how vicious the other would be at law if either of them were the first one to signal that the marriage was at an end. Thus, neither would take the step of saying, 'This marriage is finished,' because each knew that the other was so well prepared that they would be as vicious as possible. To give an example, the woman had in fact set up practice in their large private home and was running a practice which sometimes had as many as ten employees. The husband had threatened to report her to the planning authorities of his council for breach of planning regulations in running a professional practice in what was residential property. That was the level of viciousness that was going on.

Windy Dryden: Did you experience any dilemma in making such a definite statement about the end of their marriage?

Paul Brown: Well, there was the residual doubt that I had concerning the possibility that I, as therapist, was in fact bringing about the dissolution of the marriage. If one adopts the most reflective counselling style which says 'I am actually not going to, in any formal sense, be influential but am simply going to be a resource: the person has their solution within them and what they need is a sounding-board upon which to find that solution,' then that part of me was shocked to hear the other side of me which was the diagnostic clinician saying: 'On the basis of the data you have provided me then the conclusion that I reach is this.'

Windy Dryden: So you were struggling with the two major strands within you. On the one hand, the scientist practitioner who can actually address criteria to relationships and come up with statements concerning the viability . . .

Paul Brown: And in a sense can't escape those conclusions in a way that one cannot escape the conclusion that this organ has created this infection and so on . . .

Windy Dryden: And, on the other hand, the part of you that said: 'Look I am not here to make statements like that because they are potentially very influential. I am here as a resource person or one who encourages exploration.'

Paul Brown: I suppose the core of the dilemma is about being both the observer and the agent. If I hadn't said that, would there have been a different outcome? Having said that, it is now part of the experience which in a sense cannot be undone. In all forms of therapy it always seems to me to be terribly important that therapists know why they make particular interventions and have the best idea they can have of what their effects are going to be: that responses to what is happening therapeutically are not random but informed. There is always a risk in talk therapy that the therapist gets away with appearing to be doing something which is productive but actually doesn't quite know what he or she is doing. I am always encouraging both myself and my students (a) to know why we are saying something, (b) to be sure that we are in fact saying what we mean to say, and (c) to know what its effect is likely to be. Therefore, I actually do believe that what the therapist says and does is profoundly important. I can remember quite vividly when I first said, 'For these and these reasons I think your marriage is at an end,' I was quite surprised at the strength (a) with which I made the statement, and (b) of the reasons I had for making it. Its logic seemed to me to be inescapable and that it had to be said.

Windy Dryden: Going back to the model which says it is important for the therapist to know why he or she is making a response, if you act from a scientist-practitioner model you may have a different purpose than if you are operating from the psychotherapeutic model. It sounds as if some of the strain that you are experiencing here is that when you are operating from your psychotherapist 'self' you cannot completely divorce yourself from your scientist-practitioner 'self' who says: 'Wait a minute, by all the criteria that I know this is not going to work.'

Paul Brown: Yet these two aspects of oneself *have* to be integrated in a context where one still has to stay personally and therapeutically with the consequential process. Counsellors and psychotherapists don't have nurses to help bear the post-operative pain. They have to be agents of therapeutic pain *and* healers, and can't escape the consequences of their interventions.

Windy Dryden: From what you have been saying, the interesting thing is that you don't seem to experience a dilemma when your scientific-practitioner 'self' is saying: 'There is hope for this marriage on the basis of what I know about potentially good relationships.' Even though you are primarily in a therapeutic role, you don't seem to have too much problem actually making an optimistic diagnostic statement from the scientific-practitioner part of you.

Paul Brown: Because it is an optimistic one, yes. That is very interesting. The dilemma occurs when the statement to be made is apparently painful or pessimistic in nature. Yes, that is quite a productive observation. I am glad I talked to you.

DISCUSSION ISSUES

1. *Paul Brown refers to the dilemmas he experiences in attempting to integrate the 'scientist' and 'psychotherapist' parts of himself in the practice of therapy. What dilemmas (if any) do you experience in this respect? How have you attempted to resolve them?*

2. *Are you more likely to voice an opinion about the viability of a couple's marriage if you are optimistic about its future rather than pessimistic? If so, how do you account for this difference?*

3. *If you do disclose your opinion that a couple's marriage is not viable, do you think that this may hasten the end of their marriage? If so, what issues does this raise for you?*

4. *In marital therapy, do you consider that your primary responsibility is to the 'couple' or to the individuals within the couple unit? Elaborate on your view. What dilemmas do you experience in this area?*

CHAPTER ELEVEN

Confrontation or Collusion? The Dilemma of a Lonely, Burdened Behaviour Therapist

An interview with Dougal Mackay

Dougal Mackay is district top grade psychologist to Bristol and Weston Health Authority and is based at Barrow Hospital, Bristol. Despite his various administrative responsibilities, he continues to be actively involved in psychotherapy along cognitive-behavioural lines. He also holds the post of honorary lecturer in mental health at Bristol University and is currently the organizer of the psychopathology course for final-year undergraduate psychologists. In addition, he contributes to the behavioural science course for pre-clinical medical students.

He has published a number of scientific papers and review chapters on such diverse topics as sexual dysfunction, depression, insomnia, assertion problems, childhood behaviour disorders, and anxiety states. He is the author of Clinical Psychology: Theory and Therapy *(Methuen, 1975) and has co-written a self-help book entitled* Marriage and How to Survive it *(Piatkus Press, 1983). In addition to his academic and clinical publications, he has contributed to articles for such popular magazines as* Cosmopolitan *and* Company, *and broadcasts regularly on television and radio.*

He is heavily involved in the training of students from the Plymouth MSc course in clinical psychology and, indeed, regards psychotherapy supervision of trainees from all the caring professions as one of his main interests. At national level, he runs workshops on behavioural methods for the British Association for Behavioural Psychotherapy and for Psychotherapy Workshops, which he also helped to set up.

Dougal strongly advocates the behavioural analysis as the primary tool for formulating the client's problems and favours a structured, goal-oriented approach to therapy. Yet he recognizes the limitations of the behavioural model as a basis for treatment and maintains that close adherence to its theoretical principles may not always be in the best interests of his client. This he believes to be particularly so with severely depressed clients with suicidal tendencies. A particular concern of his is deciding when to implement in full the treatment programme suggested by the behavioural analysis and when to take clinical consideratons into account and pursue less ambitious goals. Since clinical manuals rarely address themselves to this issue, he feels that the responsibility for treatment planning ultimately rests with the individual therapist. This issue is explored further in the following interview.

Windy Dryden: OK, Dougal, would you like to put in your own words the dilemma you wish to talk to me about today?

Dougal Mackay: Well, Windy, as a behaviour therapist, a difficult decision I often have to make is whether or not to work directly on the problem the client presents with. I believe that we should respect the needs of our clients and do our best to help them achieve their goals. But, after carrying out a behavioural analysis of the problem, it sometimes happens that the area I would want to work on is quite different to the one the client had in mind. If I go along with him, then the chances are that my interventions will have minimal effect on the quality of his life. It may be that, according to my formulation, a direct attack on his problem will be ineffective unless other aspects of his lifestyle, for example his marriage, are worked with first. Or it could be that he is deliberately avoiding looking at the real issue but feels in need of help of some kind. Under these circumstances, to meet his request would be to collude with his defence system. But, as I say, I feel unhappy about trying to persuade a client to redefine his problem. Particularly so if this could lead to stirring up a lot of material which might prove difficult for him to deal with.

Windy Dryden: So your problem is whether to go along with the client and achieve relatively little or whether to give him a different perspective on what is really going on, with all the risks this might entail. Perhaps you could give me an example of this.

Dougal Mackay: Well, the most obvious example of this is the agoraphobic who complains that she cannot get out of the house to go to the shops. Let's say that it soon becomes clear that she is unable to assert herself with her husband and can't handle the feelings of resentment towards him. So she withdraws into herself and becomes less confident in all kinds of social situations. She dashes in and out of shops and rushes back to her house where she feels safe. After a while, even passing strangers in the street becomes a problem for her. So she goes to her doctor who tells her she has agoraphobia and prescribes tranquillizers. When this doesn't work he sends her along to me for behaviour therapy. What am I to do? I could take her out for 'walkies' as requested by both the client and the GP. I doubt if this would achieve very much but at least she wouldn't be damaged by the experience. On the other hand, I could help her to see that she is allowing her husband to trample on her and that it might be better to sort out a few things with him before tackling the phobia. With some clients this could be like opening up a can of worms. She might suddenly see the marriage as a total disaster area and that she cannot possibly be happy as long as she stays with her husband. But she can't or won't leave him because of money, the children or whatever. The next thing you know you have the husband or the doctor ringing up to accuse you of putting ideas in her head. By helping her to become fully aware of other difficult areas in her life, which she feels cannot be sorted out, I may even be interfering with her coping mechanisms and she could end up more depressed than she was before. So, although I have acted in good faith, I could be accused by all parties of having created more problems than the client came with, or thought she came with.

Windy Dryden: In these circumstances, would you consider involving the husband in therapy?

Dougal Mackay: Well I often do, but only when I feel it's really necessary. My approach is to understand the problem as fully as possible and then try to find the shortest route to achieving the goal. I don't want to create any unnecessary complications and so I only involve myself in marital or family work when it's clear that is the only way to produce change. It is the same issue really. Just as it may not always be in the client's interest to understand what the presenting problem is really about, so it may be more prudent to collude with a pathogenic system rather than to confront the members directly. In fact it can be even more risky to tinker with a family system than to challenge the individual's beliefs and assumptions. When you work with a system, you can predict some of the changes that might take place but invariably a whole series of unexpected issues arise as well. All sorts of things can happen, both inside and outside of the sessions, and, unless you have unlimited time to spend on a case, it might have been better to leave well alone.

Windy Dryden: So, when you work with more than one person it's as if, wittingly or unwittingly, you can promote change which may be out of your control. Whereas in doing individual therapy, the person with whom you have the contract is in the room with you and presumably you have more control over these changes. Is that what you're saying?

Dougal Mackay: Yes, I think that's it. I feel I've got more control over what's going on with an individual client. In dealing with two or more people, all sorts of changes can be taking place within individuals and the uncertainty factor is multiplied still further when they interact between sessions. Who knows what might be going on when they next attend? I have to say, though, that my concern to be in control over what's going on is only really a major issue when the designated client is someone who is known to be a serious suicide risk and who is only just about coping. I have a particular interest in depression and many of my clients are psychiatric inpatients who have been admitted following an overdose. It may be obvious to me that little will be achieved by working with the individual, but to involve the spouse could lead to a complete breakdown of the system. This could have devastating consequences for the designated client.

Windy Dryden: Perhaps you could provide an example which really highlights this dilemma.

Dougal Mackay: OK. At the moment I'm treating a lady of about 40 who has been admitted for depression. She has been in and out of psychiatric hospitals during the last ten years, usually following a very serious overdose. She has five adolescent children who are quite disturbed. In fact the middle child took an overdose herself last year. The husband takes no responsibility for the children, household chores, or even the finances. They are heavily in debt and he has just been made redundant. All he does, apparently, is to put his feet up, watch TV, and eat the meals that are put in front of hm. My client does all the worrying for the family and feels that she has to take responsibility for everything that could threaten the stability of the home.

Obviously I could have tackled her beliefs about being a mother through cognitive therapy, but it seemed clear to me that the family members were helping to maintain her depression. I put this to her and, although she took some persuading, she eventually allowed me to see her husband. He made it quite clear to me that he saw himself as being in no way responsible for his wife's depression. He believed that her 'illness', as he called it, was caused by hormonal changes and suggested that I got in contact with the gynaecologists who were investigating her. Given his attitude, I felt that if I persisted with my approach, he would take his anger out on the client. This would have simply reinforced the guilt-ridden, self-blaming cognitive set which was bound up with her depression. If she had then gone off and killed herself, I would have found myself in the firing line and feeling pretty guilty myself. So I cut my losses, and did some work with her to enable her to cope better with this pathogenic system. Even if I could have brought about some change in the family structure, I doubt if she would have been strong enough to handle the aggravation that would have come to the surface.

Windy Dryden: So, on the one hand, you think that if you had involved the family, not only would matters get out of your control but that this would have been damaging for your client. However, on the other hand, by not intervening with the system, I guess that might reinforce the notion that mother is the sick person in this family.

Dougal Mackay: Well that's it. You've put your finger on it. I could have come clean and said something to her husband like: 'Look whatever is going on here it's not that your wife is ill. There are some bizarre interactions going on in this family and she's the one who is coming off worst.' I didn't and, by not doing so, I was colluding with his denial of having any responsibility for her behaviour.

Windy Dryden: And also some people might argue that you are trying to help this woman adapt to a pretty destructive system.

Dougal Mackay: Well that's right and I feel very uncomfortable about being placed in that role. But what's the alternative? Actually there is an approach that can sometimes work in situations like this, although the ethics of it are somewhat debatable. What I sometimes do is to encourage the designated client to alter the system by trying out strategies we've worked on in our individual sessions. It's a bit like doing family therapy without the family. We look at what's going on at home and sort out the roles that the various members are playing in relation to each other. I then help the client to look at what would happen to these patterns of interaction if he or she were to alter his behaviour. We then work out a plan of action which we feel would disrupt the structure which is helping to maintain the problems. For this to work, the client has to learn to be assertive and, of course, patient. It takes a lot of perseverance to change a system on your own. However, if the client can see the merits of the plan, it can work.

I have to admit, though, that I feel uncomfortable about manipulating other people without their knowledge. Yet that's one way of getting round the problem you mentioned. Instead of helping the client to adjust to a pathological system, I am encouraging him to change the system from within. However this is asking a lot of the client, particularly if he or she is psychologically vulnerable to begin with.

Getting back to this issue of when to treat the individual and when to work with the system, something else which concerns me is the therapeutic contract. If I am working with just one client, then my concern is to help him to maximize his rewards without, as far as possible, infringing the rights of others. This gives me the freedom to explore any number of options. As soon as I involve the spouse or the whole family, two things happen. First, I can only deal with issues which directly relate to the system. I cannot even pursue an individual's cognitive processing errors at great length without excluding the others. The second point is that, by involving significant others as clients, I have equal responsibility to all parties. I cannot protect the interests of the designated client without forming a dishonest alliance with the others. If I continue to see the client on an individual basis in-between sessions, this can be even more confusing. Of course, I could change the nature of the contract and involve the others as co-therapists, but this would be another way of colluding with the 'sick role' game. So, as I see it, there are disadvantages as well as advantages when considering whether or not to work with the system, even if the family members are willing to be involved.

Windy Dryden: So it's a question of who your contract is with. In the case of individual therapy that's clear. If an individual client comes along then your contract is with that person. One might argue though that since, if that person is in a relationship, any internal changes that occur have an impact on the other people involved so that the responsibility issue is not quite cut and dried. However, when you are seeing two people, are your clients the two individuals or the relationship?

Dougal Mackay: In behavioural marital therapy, the client is the relationship. By this I mean that I am working with maladaptive patterns of interactions which both parties contribute to equally. My task is to analyse these sequences, help them to become aware of the part each person plays in maintaining them, and encourage them to approach the change process in a spirit of collaborative endeavour. So I'm only concerned with beliefs and behaviour which are bound up with the difficulties in the relationship. They may well each have similar problems in other areas of their lives but these would not appear on the agenda of behavioural marital or family therapy. So what I am saying is that, in individual therapy, there is the freedom to explore cognitions in as much depth as both I and the client want to, and we can scan across all aspects of his life in our attempt to maximize rewards and decrease costs.

Windy Dryden: And that leads you to say that you are less circumscribed in individual therapy?

Dougal Mackay: That's right. There's a sort of paradox here. I am less circumscribed in individual therapy and have more control over what's going on. In marital or family work, I have to stick to a much tighter agenda but have less control over the situation. My interventions can lead to a whole host of unexpected consequences.

Perhaps I can give another clinical example to illustrate this dilemma. A client was referred to me recently with a public-speaking phobia. In order to succeed in his job, he needed to be able to address large meetings. From the behavioural analysis, it emerged that the public-speaking problem was just one manifestation of a more generalized state of unassertiveness. So I proceeded to analyse this and found that his wife was, wittingly or unwittingly, punishing him for standing up for himself. Her attacks on him made him feel guilty, repentant, and so on. It seemed clear that, so long as she persisted in doing this, he would remain unassertive and therefore unlikely to perform well in the public-speaking situation. I also got the impression that he would get much more out of life if his level of self-confidence increased. So I invited his wife to attend and started them off on marital therapy. As soon as he was able to air his grievances, she decided she had had enough of the relationship and bang, off she went.

As you can imagine, this left him completely devastated. He's still got his phobia and he's blaming me for the break-up of his marriage: 'I came with a public-speaking phobia and all you've done is to wreck my marriage.' And yet, in good faith, I had embarked on the treatment programme which seemed most appropriate for his particular problem. I honestly didn't think that a relaxation tape and some coping strategies would have much effect, unless the marital system had been tackled in the first place. So, where I help the client to redefine his problem and tackle a different issue than the one he wanted help with, it's difficult to say I've done a good job when it all goes wrong for him. Privately I might feel that the break-up of the marriage was the best thing that could have happened to him but the point is that he was unable to see it that way.

So I suppose that, after experiences like that, I hesitate before interfering with systems. As I see it, such action is only warranted if (a) it is totally justifiable from the analysis, and (b) if I am convinced, having met the spouse or family, that there is a sound basis for a treatment alliance which is likely to lead to something constructive for everyone. However, even so, there are still risks. You never know what accidental damage you might cause. It's a bit like surgery isn't it? A good surgeon favours conservative methods of treatment wherever possible and takes up his scalpel only when it is absolutely necessary. That sums up my feelings about working with systems as opposed to individuals.

Windy Dryden: Could it be that the behavioural perspective which you take on clinical matters doesn't particularly help you to anticipate the unintended consequences that occur when you do involve other people in the system?

Dougal Mackay: Well, let me think about that one. I think the difficulty here is that, in behaviour therapy, it's impossible to fully assess a marriage or family without making certain interventions. So if, after three sessions, I decide it's not a good idea to proceed, it may be too late. Bang! These unforeseen consequences have occurred and there's no way I can pull out now. So I don't think my model lets me down. I can't think of a better way of predicting outcome than collecting data systematically and formulating hypotheses. As I see it, not many models do this. The trouble is that the behavioural analysis enables my clients, as well as myself, to pinpoint the trouble spots. And remember they have plenty of opportunity to take things further between sessions. So, by the time I've got a clear idea of the risks involved in pursuing treatment, they may have already got there ahead of me. So, if anything, the behavioural approach is perhaps too effective at helping clients to see what is really going on. With an unstructured approach, presumably the dangers are far less.

Windy Dryden: So, is it tempting for you to say that as a result of the risks involved in working with the system, you should confine yourself to the individual?

Dougal Mackay: No I wouldn't go as far as that. In fact, I can remember another public-speaking phobic I worked with—this was just after I qualified—who made tremendous progress as a result of assertion training. I had been seeing him on an individual basis and never thought to involve his wife. However, he changed so much as a result of my interventions that his wife couldn't cope with his level of assertion and got put on anti-depressants by her doctor. You can't win, can you? What I do these days is to see the client's partner as a matter of course, before starting treatment. My approach is usually something like: 'I would like you to come along to help me sort out what kind of treatment might be most appropriate for your partner.' This is sometimes a bit of a 'con', because I may already have reached the opinion that it's primarily a marital problem. But there are many other reasons why I might want to have some sort of relationship with the spouse.

After we have met up, there are a number of options open to me. I might think: 'Yes, it really is a marital problem and he or she sees it that way as well.' If the client does as well, then there's no problem. Or I may conclude that the system is contributing to the presenting difficulty but decide that it's a real can of worms and best left alone. For example, if they're both in their sixties and have had a problem marriage for forty years, why stir things up at this late stage unless you have a very good reason to? Again, if my analysis or, dare I say it, my intuition tells me that it's a troubled relationship, I wouldn't proceed if I reckoned that my client would be worse off out of that system. I would leave the marriage well alone and con-centrate on coping strategies through individual therapy.

Another possibility is enlisting the help of the partner as co-therapist, as I mentioned earlier. However, I don't feel very happy about doing this because it suggests that I see one of them as 'well' and the other as 'ill'. Finally, I could offer therapy to the non-designated client, if he or she is having difficulty in coping with the partner's behaviour. I would say some-thing like: 'You seem very distressed as well and it's clear to me that what's been happening recently has had quite an effect on you. Would you find it useful to come along for some help?' I don't do this very often because, by seeing them both separately, I am setting up a potential game situation. So, I've no hard-and-fast rules about individual and marital therapy. All I'm saying is that, since most of my clients are very vulnerable people, I need a lot of convincing before embarking on marital or family therapy.

Windy Dryden: From the way you have spoken today, it seems as if *you* are very much in charge of the therapeutic decision-making. It is you who decides whether to see a person individually and it is you who will decide whether the person is to be a therapeutic aide or a fully participating member of a conjoint therapy. Is my impression accurate?

Dougal Mackay: Well that's true to some degree. I would find it very difficult to say to a potential suicide: 'Look, it's quite clear that it's your marriage which is making you depressed. Do you think we should try to work something out there? However, it could all blow up in our faces and you find yourself alone before you know what's happened.' Obviously I would never put it like that but what do you do? With a *vulnerable* client, I think it would be quite unethical for me to spell out my formulation and lead him to suggest a course of action which could possibly have very damaging consequences for him. What I usually do, when faced with this issue, is to hint that some conjoint work could be useful. I might say something like: 'I get the impression that your partner's behaviour is not making it easy for you to cope. Do you think it might be helpful if we met up as a threesome to discuss some of these points?' The client can then decide whether or not to take up this option. The key point here is that if he says no, I will drop the matter, whatever my private views, at least for the time being. By adopting such a low-key approach, I hopefully prevent the client from having to question assumptions which he isn't yet ready to look at. OK, it may mean that our goals have to be limited but, but with my vulnerable clients, I would rather be safe than sorry.

Windy Dryden: So what role does the client or the client's spouse play in therapeutic decision-making?

Dougal Mackay: Well, as I say, I may try to protect the suicidal client from additional stress by not putting the issue to him as openly and honestly as I would wish to. If I don't spell out the options then obviously he is not involved in decision-making at all. Looking at it the other way around, if the designated client suggested to me that it was basically a marital problem, then I would want him to convince me that my analysis was incomplete. He could, after all, be scapegoating his partner when basically the *primary* problem was his and his alone. Just the other week, for example, a retired male client tried to persuade me that his wife was the cause of all his unhappiness. He said that she played golf all the time and took no account of his needs. When I saw her, it turned out that she played once a week and only at times which fitted in with his plans. She apparently put herself out for him in all sorts of other ways and clearly had tried to make the relationship work.

I then decided to see them both and, from that interview, formed the strong impression that I was dealing with a case of pathological jealousy. He couldn't bear to have her out of his sight and was unwilling to negotiate any compromise which would lead to her having any private life of her own. Although she was perfectly willing to come along, I felt that it would be more useful to take him on alone, at least to start with. As you can imagine, it wasn't easy to get across to him the reason why I thought that individual therapy was more appropriate. However he did go along with my opinion—somewhat reluctantly I have to admit—and was eventually able to soften his belief that his wife, if she really loved him, should want to spend all her time with him. It worked out all right in the end and they were both pleased with the results. But I have to admit that I had the major say as to the kind of therapy we undertook. From the behavioural analysis, that seemed to me to be the most cost-effective way of dealing with the problem.

Windy Dryden: So what about the client's spouse? Does he or she have any say in the matter?

Dougal Mackay: Well, if I'm honest, not a lot. My primary responsibility is to the person who is formally referred to me. If my client wants individual treatment, and I believe that that is the best way of proceeding, I would not allow his partner to persuade me otherwise. I have to say that that rarely happens, thank goodness. When it does, I usually offer the spouse the option of therapy or support of some kind on the assumption that he or she is seeking help.

So I suppose I have to admit that I have more of a say about the form therapy will take than either of the other two parties. I hope I haven't given the impression that my clients and I are in a constant state of conflict about what should be done. It's pretty rare to have a disagreement of this kind but it can be difficult to deal with when it does arise. But, as I see it, my main task is to decide what is the most cost-effective treatment for the person who comes for help, always bearing in mind what I think he can handle.

Windy Dryden: Let's get back to your main dilemma. You feel that if you treat the individual, when you believe that the system is pathogenic, you are colluding with the notion that your client is the 'sick' member. Yet, if you try to persuade the client to embark on marital or family work, it could all blow up in your face. Is that right?

Dougal Mackay: Yes, that's the big issue as I see it. Going back to the case of the public-speaking phobic whom I talked into marital therapy, it could hardly be considered a success. He more or less said to me: 'You told me that involving my wife was the right thing to do. But it proved devastating to me and, even if the marriage wasn't up to much, I wish you'd kept your hands off it and just worked on the phobia. I would rather be in a dud marriage than be totally isolated.' Personally I felt that he was better off out of that marriage and would have liked to have kept him in treatment but, after that fiasco, he wanted out. He felt he had trusted me and that I had let him down. So there are big risks involved when you work with systems and I need some convincing before I attempt to modify relationships.

Windy Dryden: It's almost like the government warning on the side of your cigarette packet, where Dougal says 'Therapy may be bad for your relationship.' In a sense, that is a joke but there is a serious part to it. To what extent do we as therapists honestly say that we are entering somewhat uncharted waters here and, if we look at your relationship, one of the consequences might well be that the relationship may come to an end as a result?

Dougal Mackay: Not often enough I suspect. What it boils down to is whether or not it is our duty to open up people's eyes to enable them to see clearly what is going on—no matter how painful or devastating this might be. Who are we to insist on playing the truth game when our clients, who are ultimately responsible for their own destinies, have chosen not to? To be cynical for a moment, if all we do is to help the damaged person to move from one pathological system to social isolation, or possibly to another 'sick' system, then can we justify the distress and upheaval we have caused him and the many others who are involved? I just think we should be more careful when contemplating action which, although indicated by our models, has all kinds of unpredictable consequences for the person concerned.

Windy Dryden: Another debating point is: 'Who is responsible for making these choices and for whom?'

Dougal Mackay: That's right. We know only too well that, as therapists, the very way in which we present our formulation affects the way the client comes to see his difficulties. A subtle change of emphasis here and there and he can be convinced that family therapy is the only answer. The frightening thing is that we can be so influenced by our theoretical orientations that we don't even recognize that all we are presenting is one version of 'the truth' rather than an objective appraisal of the situation. I personally think that the behavioural analysis is less value-laden than most other forms of psychotherapeutic assessment, but I am kidding myself if I believe it to be anything other than a set of hypotheses. And even if I could prove, in some way, that my formulations are always factually correct, am I justified in sharing this knowledge with a client who may not be able to cope with it?

Windy Dryden: Right, to conclude, I think you are nicely illustrating that, although behaviour therapy prides itself in terms of the application of scientific principles, there is no way in which behaviour therapists, or any other therapists, can keep values out of the therapeutic enterprise.

Dougal Mackay: We are fooling ourselves if we think otherwise and, during the course of therapy, there are any number of choice-points . . .

Windy Dryden: Where empirical data may not help us?

Dougal Mackay: Absolutely right. Choice-points where the therapist's attitudes and beliefs—both personal and theoretical—affect how he feeds back information to the client. No matter how expert you may be in a particular form of therapy, you can't get round this. But what concerns me most of all is where we are so 'hung up' on our models, that we force 'insights' on to the client which he would rather not know about.

Let me end this interview with a summary of my position. My role, as I see it, is to devise the most cost-effective programme for enabling the client to achieve his goal. Sometimes, however, my analysis tells me that the problem is much more complicated than the client thinks it is and that, to *really* help him, I need to reframe it for him in my terms. If I am being true to my model, that's what I should do. However he may not thank me for persuading him that he is less adequate as a person than he thought he was or that his marriage is a bit of a sham. Added to this, if I break down his defences or expose the flaws in his marital relationships, there is no guarantee that he will benefit from this experience. In fact, by involving his wife or family, I may end up causing considerable distress to other people as well. I'm not saying that we should always play it safe and go along with the client's perceptions of his problem. I couldn't do this job if I spent most of my time supporting sick systems or working on pseudo-problems. The difficulty is knowing when to confront and when to collude. The textbooks don't have the answers and, in the end, the decision has to be mine. It's a very lonely position to be in when you have such responsibility for other people's lives and, when it comes to it, have to rely on your own personal judgment. So that's my dilemma.

Windy Dryden: So one might sum up by saying that yours is the dilemma of a lonely burdened behaviour therapist.

Dougal Mackay: Yes, I'll settle for that.

DISCUSSION ISSUES

1. *Under what conditions might you choose to confront clients with the full implications of their problems and under what conditions might you choose to protect them from these implications? What factors influence your decisions in this respect?*
2. *When might you choose to work in the arena of individual therapy and help a client cope with a pathogenic family system and when might you involve that system in therapy? What criteria do you employ in making such decisions?*
3. *Dougal Mackay reports experiencing a sense of discomfort in helping clients in individual therapy alter a family system by encouraging them to experiment with different behaviours in that system. He considers that he is helping to manipulate other people without their knowledge. What dilemmas (if any) do you have about this strategy?*
4. *What dilemmas do you experience in working directly with marital and family systems?*
5. *When do you make unilateral decisions in therapy and when do you involve your clients in the decision-making process? What dilemmas do you experience in this area?*

CHAPTER TWELVE

Death by Starvation: Whose Decision?

An interview with Fay Fransella

Fay Fransella is director of the Centre for Personal Construct Psychology and emeritus reader in clinical psychology at the University of London. In 1982 she founded the first centre to focus totally on the theory and application of personal construct psychology. This was to meet the demand for teaching and services which comes mainly from non-psychologists.

Since the late 1960s she has played an active role as teacher, researcher, author and psychotherapist in making the work of George Kelly known internationally.

Her major research work has been concerned with the development of a personal construct theoretical model to account for stuttering. She then tested this model in a programme of treatment research described in her book Personal Change and Reconstruction: Research on a Treatment of Stuttering *(Academic Press, 1972). Since then further research for the Department of Health and Social Security followed up some of the findings relating to relapse after treatment.*

Her other major area of research has been in the field of weight disorders—both obesity and anorexia nervosa. She was interested in applying the model stemming from the stuttering research, that any form of behaviour adopted by a person over a long period of time will come to have a profound effect on how that person construes the 'self'. She argues that it is only by building up a picture of another 'self' that is a fluent person or someone of 'normal' weight that one can move from the undesired to the desired state.

Although she has carried out research into both weight extremes, her psychotherapeutic and counselling work has largely been concerned with the obese person. The reason for this biased emphasis is her reluctance to treat someone who is resistant to such interventions. The anorexic girl typically comes for treatment to satisfy some-one else's wish rather than her own. Fay feels that such a situation runs counter to the basic philosophy of personal construct theory and yet realizes that the anorexic girl may well need help in spite of her feelings to the contrary. This theme is explored further in the following interview.

Windy Dryden: OK, Fay, would you like to tell me what your dilemma is?

Fay Fransella: Well, the one that exercises my mind most at the moment is whether I have the right to intervene with a client who actually doesn't want my help; such as young people suffering from anorexia nervosa.

Windy Dryden: So, on the one hand they don't seek help and on the other?

Fay Fransella: On the other, at the end of the road, there is death in the extreme case. However, everything that I and some others like me stand for is the notion that individuals are responsible for themselves. Thus, if they say, 'I don't want your help,' you should not intervene. And yet I know that without help of some sort, unless there is some spontaneous improvement, the young person is never going to have any form of what I would call a 'happy life', because they are going to become more and more obsessed with the problem. I have usually found them to be most unhappy people. That is the dilemma as I see it.

Windy Dryden: Is someone who is anorexic free enough from emotional disturbance to make a decision that might be in their best interest?

Fay Fransella: My immediate reaction is to say 'yes'. But it depends what you mean by emotional disturbance. I see what you are getting at; that they are so bound up in their 'problem' that they can't see that they actually need help. However they *can* see that they don't want it, which to me implies that they have an idea what it is about. It's not that they're passive—like someone who has, for instance, been shut away in a hen-house for the whole of their childhood and who is not able to tell you that he would rather not be in a hen-house because he has no experience of anything else. I wouldn't be fussed at all about intervening in that case. But these young people do seem to have made what to them is a rational choice. And yet we do intervene.

Windy Dryden: Why do we intervene?

Fay Fransella: I suppose for two reasons. First, because there is social pressure. They come because a doctor says they must or their parents say they must. Second, and more fundamental, because there is the potential threat that they will starve themselves to death. Now, I'm sure that this is not their aim. But it can be the end result. In personal construct theory there is a notion which states that people with a problem can be seen as being 'stuck'. In a way, these young people are personally 'stuck', because they can't see outside their current constricted view of the world. It could therefore be argued that it is a good thing to try and give them the opportunity to see outside it.

But if you succeed in helping them see alternative ways of construing the world other than through thinness, and they then relapse, you are in an even worse situation. They have seen the outside world and have decided that it is not as good as their present one—so they return to the old familiar one where it is uncomfortable but safe.

What is coming up for me is a notion that people *should* be helped to have opportunities for personal development. The more I talk about it the more I don't like it because personal construct theory is so dead against any value judgment like that.

Windy Dryden: So, you also come into conflict with personal construct theory over this issue?

Fay Fransella: That does seem to be so. Personal construct theory and certainly Kelly's philosophy state that the person has created themselves. There are no prescriptions that this is a good way to construe or that is a bad way. It depends whether it is OK for the individual. If it serves the individual's purposes then we, as interveners, have no right to say: 'You should be different.' Of course, we do that when we say, 'You have committed a crime,' or 'You have injured that person.' But that is a bit different. That is society saying we have certain norms of behaviour and we must obey those norms. However, these girls have not done anything against society.

Windy Dryden: So the one pressure on you is the social pressure?

Fay Fransella: That's a minimal pressure. One can always say to mum: 'Sorry, there is nothing I can do for your daughter.'

Windy Dryden: And the other pressure?

Fay Fransella: The GPs or psychiatrists who say: 'We have tried drugs, we have tried hospital treatment and we have told her if she doesn't decide to put on weight soon she will be spending the rest of her life going in and out of hospital. Can you see what you can do with her?' That is a terrible moral pressure.

Windy Dryden: So, it sounds as if you are choosing between the lesser of two evils. If you don't intervene then that person has a very unhappy life ahead of them, but if you do intervene you violate a principle which you and construct theory hold dear.

Fay Fransella: Yes, basically because the individual is not being treated as if they are their own master. What GPs and psychiatrists want to do is reasonable—that is, to save the girl's life. They have to do whatever they see fit within this perspective of saving life. I don't see an alternative. And yet I don't like such interventions. I think one *can* help some of these girls; but first of all you have to persuade them that they need help. And that is manipulation.

Windy Dryden: And from your point of view what is so bad about manipulation in this context?

Fay Fransella: What I don't like is that I am setting out to do something without that person's consent. Personal construct psychotherapy is about finding out where the person is at the present and helping that person find alternative ways of construing their present position. However, before I can start doing that with the anorexic girl I have to get her into the frame of mind that she *wants* to explore her present position. Consequently, I have to persuade her, in a very real sense, to my way of thinking.

Windy Dryden: I guess we are talking about a situation where the person isn't free to vote with their feet in the sense of not turning up for appointments. They are under an obligation to come because they are under threat of something nasty happening to them if they don't come and see you.

Fay Fransella: That's an interesting point because, in a sense, I suppose they are free not to come. Most are over eighteen and at the end of the day no-one can *force* you to spend your life in hospital if you do not want to. So, in the extreme, I suppose you are right. She can say no. A good point. I feel better already!

Windy Dryden: In what sense?

Fay Fransella: She does have a choice even though the pressures on her are very great and she is not usually very old. She *can* leave home or some alternative massive thing like that.

Windy Dryden: So if they are over the age of legal consent that helps you to solve the dilemma?

Fay Fransella: I think it's a bit of a help.

Windy Dryden: But when they are not over that age?

Fay Fransella: Then the dilemma is still there. It is not like school phobia; the child has to go to school because the parents are legally bound to send them. There is no law that says you have to eat.

Windy Dryden: You could act, as I said before, in a 'hostile' fashion (in Kellyan terms) by refusing to have anything to do with the issue and therefore maintaining your stance that it is the individual's right to determine his or her own destiny.

Fay Fransella: Yes, but I do feel that they need help and that some of them can be helped to get out of their predicament and so lead a more 'normal' life. If I or someone else does not do all they can to help them, then it's back to a life of hospitals or they may even face some more radical medical treatment.

Windy Dryden: You seem to be wrestling with, on the one hand, being true to a principle that you really hold dear and, on the other hand, if you do hold to that principle the individual suffers.

Fay Fransella: Potentially yes. There are some penalties to that position. My dilemma is wrestling with Kelly's psychological and philosophical principles in these instances.

Windy Dryden: What would your experience be if you violate one of these principles?

Fay Fransella: What I now find interesting is that I very rarely take on these people for treatment. I have done research into anorexia nervosa, but when it comes to therapy I ask a colleague to undertake it. So I side-step my own dilemma.

Windy Dryden: It doesn't solve it for you, but it shelves it for you.

Fay Fransella: Yes.

Windy Dryden: Let me push you here and let's suppose that there is nobody around for you to refer to, and you receive a request to see an under-legal-aged girl who is quite seriously anorexic and who doesn't want to seek help from you. In other words you can't really dodge the issue. Where would that leave you?

Fay Fransella: I have no doubt that I would see her. What I am not totally sure about is whether or not I would be 'hostile' with that person and 'prove' that I could not persuade her to be helped. I would then be able to say: 'Well, there you are, I always knew it was no good trying to help these young people.' That would be a good example of pure 'hostility'.

Windy Dryden: Would your awareness of this possibility help you avoid that situation?

Fay Fransella: I am not convinced that if you know about something then you can guard against it. To persuade the girl that it may be worthwhile to explore her present position really does take every ounce of concentration because you have to try to work within her own construing system. You have only got to keep back a vestige of your own construing system not to do the job well.

Windy Dryden: Could you envisage a strategy whereby you actually share your dilemma with this person, and that actually forms the basis of your therapy? You might actually say to this person, 'Look, I have been asked to see you, I am uneasy about it, I am uneasy about it for these reasons,' and you spell out your reasons to the person: that on the one hand you believe that people have a free choice and yet you are aware that the consequences of her continuing to starve herself would be either death or harsh treatment. Consequently, you have that person help you with your dilemma.

Fay Fransella: Yes, but we are talking about a 15 year-old girl. I suppose I don't have enough experience of 15 year-olds to know how they would take that. But that seems to be quite a hefty thing to put to a 15 year-old girl, doesn't it?

Windy Dryden: As is giving them the responsibility to kill themselves.

Fay Fransella: Yes, but that's not how they see it. They don't see that as a possible end result. They are not committing suicide, not in their own terms, I am sure.

Windy Dryden: So you would doubt whether that particular strategy would work?

Fay Fransella: It is a strategy I have used in other contexts. I am not against the strategy as such. It is a perfectly legitimate way of proceeding in therapy. Whether or not it would work with a 15 year-old girl I have my doubts.

Windy Dryden: So, if we discount that strategy and if we discount your 'hostile' strategy, then what's left?

Fay Fransella: Back to the drawing board. There are always alternative ways of construing any event. However, sometimes people can be trapped by their ways of construing the events in their environment. So we are back to where we started. We *can* say that we know what's best for them at a particular time, but it is more than possible that *they* are doing what they see as best for them at that particular time. So you end up by saying: 'I've better knowledge than you have. I have a wider view of the world my girl! If you would only stop being so silly you can grow up, become a woman and go out and have experience of all that life as a woman has to offer you. Life will open up before you.'

Windy Dryden: So, no matter which way you turn you cannot help but violate a Kellyan principle.

Fay Fransella: Maybe I can try and find another Kellyan principle that makes it OK. I think that what I am talking about here is a very superordinate construct and maybe it is too superordinate and I need to bring it more down to earth— to a more practical level. I would intervene to help people come off drugs, even if the person didn't want to, because it is so clearly not in that person's best interest.

Windy Dryden: And how do you solve that dilemma for yourself?

Fay Fransella: Perhaps by never having actually worked with those who are addicted to drugs!

Windy Dryden: You mean you *would* do that?

Fay Fransella: Yes, I would. I would see no problem because they are so obviously damaging themselves physically and psychologically under the influence of drugs and are not fully capable of taking a rational decision.

Windy Dryden: Although one could argue that that is exactly the position with the anorexic.

Fay Fransella: One could but I don't see it like that. I find it very difficult to see it that way. When you talk to anorexic girls they seem to have it quite clearly worked out that this is the way for them. Now I could take a leaf out of Hilda Bruch's book and say that they are deluded; that really they have a false belief that they are very fat, even though the reality is that they are only 6½ stone.

Windy Dryden: Well, that might actually help you to solve the dilemma.

Fay Fransella: It would help me to solve the dilemma if I actually believed it. It depends on what one means by a delusion. If they do indeed see themselves as totally different from the way the majority of people see them, then that would be called a delusion. But I am not absolutely convinced that this is so. I have done some work on body image and certainly these girls do overestimate their body size, but so do a great many other groups including many women of 'normal' weight, pregnant women and even some obese women.

Windy Dryden: I am reminded from what you say of that joke about Carl Rogers, where he is working with a patient who says: 'Well, Dr Rogers, this is the last time I will be see you because I am going to commit suicide.' Rogers reflects the patient's feelings and the patient opens the window and says, 'OK, Dr Rogers, I am leaving,' and Rogers gives another reflection whereupon the patient jumps out of the window and Rogers looks out of the window and says 'Plop', reflecting to the very end. Well, in reality Rogers has talked about that and said, 'Look, in no way would I have allowed that person to jump. I would have stopped that person,' and, asked why, he responded: 'Because a strong feeling would have bubbled up and led me to take action.'

Fay Fransella: So you are saying one makes a distinction between one's theoretical framework and one's personal strategy or beliefs?

Windy Dryden: Right. I think it is true to say that a lot of people in Britain do respect you and your work, but one criticism that I have heard a couple of times is that you overly identify yourself with Kellyan principles. I am sensing that in a way here too.

Fay Fransella: I certainly find them a useful philosophical framework through which to conduct my life.

Windy Dryden: And yet that might conflict with the strong sort of personal feeling which when looked at closely may violate one of these principles.

Fay Fransella: Yes. And this is perfectly possible within the theoretical system itself. When one is actually being a therapist or counsellor I do believe that to be professional it is important that you have a framework within which you work, one which gives you guidance through the complexities of another's experience. This dilemma is produced when these principles and those guiding 'me as a person' come together. At the end of the day, I do see anorexic girls and do my best to help them. At the end of the day I, as a person, win as opposed to the Kellyan principles. As I pointed out, if I really adhered to these I would say no.

Windy Dryden: So although the dilemma doesn't go away you are not paralysed.

Fay Fransella: I am not paralysed because I do act. Every time it comes up I am consciously aware of the conflict. Perhaps I am misreading Kelly's notions. Perhaps I am using it too rigidly and in too pure a fashion. Because he does say we all obviously create ourselves within certain contexts and that these contexts or environments are in part created by the society and culture within which we live.

Windy Dryden: How do you think Kelly would have resolved this dilemma? Do you think he would have resolved it in the same way as you?

Fay Fransella: If he were to have had the same dilemma I think he might. Certainly his extreme humanity shone through strongly.

Windy Dryden: Does that comfort you in a way?

Fay Fransella: No, I don't think so. I don't feel the need for comfort in that sense. Or support. I am aware of the dilemma. You have helped me to spell it out. It hasn't resolved it. It is still there. In a sense I find that good. You have helped me make a useful distinction and one on which I will dwell. One can never fully live a theory or a philosophical principle. At the end of the day, I am 'me'.

DISCUSSION ISSUES

1. *Under what conditions (if any) do you intervene with 'clients' who do not want your help? What dilemmas do you experience in this respect?*
2. *What criteria do you use in determining whether clients are responsible for making appropriate judgments concerning their welfare?*

3. *To what extent do you find that becoming aware of your dilemmas as a therapist helps you to resolve them? If awareness is insufficient in this respect, what other factors do you find personally helpful?*

4. *Which of your clients have led you to experience therapeutic dilemmas? What were these dilemmas and how (if relevant) did you resolve them?*

5. *Which of your personal beliefs lead you into conflict with your therapeutic orientation? What dilemmas do you experience in this regard?*

CHAPTER THIRTEEN

The Non-improving Patient

An interview with Paul Wachtel

Paul L. Wachtel is professor of psychology and associate director of the PhD programme in clinical psychology at City College and the Graduate Center of the City University of New York. He received his PhD from Yale in the days when both John Dollard and Neal Miller were active members of the faculty and this undoubtedly played a role in his later efforts to contribute to the integration of psychodynamic and behavioural points of view. Upon leaving Yale, however, he immersed himself primarily in mastering the psychoanalytic point of view, receiving psychoanalytic training in the post-doctoral programme in psychoanalysis and psychotherapy at New York University.

After a few years of doing research on attention and cognitive styles at the Downstate Medical Center in New York, Paul's psychoanalytic interests led him to the Research Center for Mental Health at NYU where, under the leadership of George Klein and Robert Holt, a team of impressive clinician-researchers had been assembled. His participation in the critical examination of psychoanalytic assumptions at the Research Center led him in a different direction than most of his colleagues— first to an increasing respect for the underestimated contributions of Karen Horney and Harry Stack Sullivan and then to a recognition of ways in which their reformulations of psychoanalytic thought provided a path toward incorporating new developments from other therapeutic approaches.

Over the last dozen years at City College Paul has worked toward developing an integrative approach to psychotherapy and personality theory, described in his book Psychoanalysis and Behavior Therapy *(Basic Books, 1977) and in numerous papers and chapters since. He has also been actively engaged in psychologically oriented* social criticism, particularly in explicating the psychological costs of a growth- and consumer-oriented way of life. His recent book, The Poverty of Affluence (Free Press, 1983), is a comprehensive exploration of those costs, as well as a sympathetic but critical examination of efforts (such as the human potential movement and the counterculture of the 1960s) to point toward a psychologically oriented alternative and a pointed exposure of the fallacies of those, like Christopher Lasch, who claimed simplistically that those efforts were 'narcissistic'.

The interview that follows can be seen as a reflection of the two major concerns which have occupied Paul over the years—the practice of psychotherapy and the values and ethical issues that are all too frequently omitted from psychological discourse.

Windy Dryden: Could you phrase the dilemma you wish to talk about in your own words.

Paul Wachtel: The dilemma is one that actually derives from the way you phrased what this book is all about. Namely that therapy is often described as if it was always effective and yet the fact is that no therapist is universally effective. It is not as uncommon as I would wish for me to have the experience that although the patient does develop a relationship with me as therapist, he or she does not seem to benefit from therapy with me. In these instances I may conclude that the person would do better with someone else and feel some ethical qualms about continuing to take the person's money or use up his or her therapeutic time when the person could be working with someone else. And yet if I share this thought with the patient he or she may feel hurt or rejected. I think this is a dilemma that many therapists must experience.

Windy Dryden: So, on the one hand you consider that therapy isn't working and yet on the other hand you feel that the person may become more psychologically disturbed as a result of you actually expressing this concern.

Paul Wachtel: Right. The very fact that a relationship has been established between myself and the patient means that all my actions have consequences and as a lot of research has shown, therapy can be for better or worse. Thus if I confront the patient with my feeling that what we are doing may not be helpful to him, this very act may in itself be harmful. The patient may come to feel that, 'Here is one more failure in my life,' or 'This person does not like me or would rather be with someone else.' So, dealing with this issue raises a lot of questions.

Windy Dryden: Can you say a little more about what the dilemmas are for you in actually dealing with this issue with patients?

Paul Wachtel: Well, one of the dilemmas is that if we as therapists are honest with ourselves, we tend to enjoy working with patients who are responsive to the way we work more than with patients who are not responsive. We like the person better who seems really to gain from the therapeutic experience. This compounds the problem because the very patient we are discussing here is often the patient we do not like as much. It might not initially have been that way and it may not have anything to do with the intrinsic qualities of the patient, but the very fact that you have worked with someone who is not reinforcing you—by improving—can make that person less appealing. Therefore when the patient thinks that you as therapist want to get rid of him because you don't like him as much as your other patients there is an element of truth to this suspicion. It is not the truth as *he* sees it, since this situation has not developed because of his intrinsic qualities, but the therapist does have to deal with the fact that the patient is picking up on something real.

Windy Dryden: So you come to dislike the person not for his intrinsic qualities, but because therapy isn't going as well as you would like.

Paul Wachtel: Yes, because I am frustrated by the experience. Or at the very least—because it is hard for me even in this self-revelatory situation to quite face the sense of disliking the patient—that I like the patient less than I might like other patients. I might add that part of the reason that I phrase this in such a hedging way is that the people that I am talking about often have attractive personalities. They are by no means necessarily obnoxious or uninteresting. The frustration—the lack of therapeutic liking, if you will—comes from the fact that for whatever reason they are not changing very much even though they want to.

Windy Dryden: Are we only talking about patients who are not changing or does this situation also apply to patients who are getting worse?

Paul Wachtel: Well, in some sense when a patient is getting worse it can actually be less discouraging, because you have the sense that whatever is going on has at least had some impact and there are often possibilities to reverse the trend. In this case there is a sense of variability. What is even harder is the person who simply stays unchanged.

Windy Dryden: With the patient who stays the same, I guess you are faced with the choice of continuing therapy and not affecting the patient or of raising the issue of his not improving and the patient deteriorating as a result of you raising it.

Paul Wachtel: Exactly. I think some therapists can ward off this dilemma by adopting the view that therapy is a long process that can take many years before the patient exhibits some improvement. This view states that the changes have to be internal and subtle before they can become manifest. This is a useful defence for these therapists to adopt. My own belief about the process of therapy is that if it does not start having some kind of impact fairly soon, I am not optimistic about the likelihood of movement later on, whether we are talking about brief or long-term therapy. The best prognosis whether someone will change as a result of therapy is whether they begin to show early signs of change. These early signs have an impact in their daily lives which feed back and produce further change. This point of view leads me in some sense to become impatient with the therapeutic process rather than be sanguine and sit back and hope that something will occur some time in the distant future.

Windy Dryden: How have you attempted to deal with this dilemma in the past?

Paul Wachtel: A lot of soul-searching and wrestling with the issue is part of it—a preliminary stage, if you will. However, I try to find a way to confront the issue as a shared issue between the patient and myself. I don't view it as a case of patient 'resistance' but as something that the two of us are participating in. I try to present the impasse not as a sign of the patient's failure but as an inappropriate matching of two people. This view is more interactional in nature than that customarily adopted by traditional analytic therapists.

Windy Dryden: Do you ever discuss with patients, at the outset of therapy, the possibility that such an impasse might occur later?

Paul Wachtel: I have done so, on occasion, when I feel somehow apprehensive about whether therapy is going to work. When I sense this, I will at the outset make it clear that there will be a trial period to see if we can work together, to see whether I am the right therapist for this particular person. In doing so I try to get over the point that I won't be hurt if we conclude that we cannot productively work together. This is important because often the patient may feel concerned about hurting the therapist. The patient feels protective towards the therapist in the same way as children are often very protective towards their parents. Many psychological problems that bring people to therapy have involved the patient adopting a distressful position in order not to confront the way a parent has let them down. This often occurs with their therapists also. So I stress that my self-esteem does not depend on my being able to cure every single person that comes to me for help.

Windy Dryden: Do your raise this issue routinely with patients at the outset of therapy?

Paul Wachtel: No, because there are some people who have been raised by parents who have spent a lot of time warning them about the terrors of the world, warning them about what could go wrong and how dangerous things are. With such patterns, my raising this issue at the outset would be counter-productive. Franz Alexander's[1] undervalued concept of the 'corrective emotional experience' is important here. This viewpoint states that if therapy is going to be helpful then the therapist has to present a *different* kind of relationship than the patient has had with his parents. So if I were to raise this caveat at the outset of therapy with such patients I may be showing them once more that the world is a dangerous place where things may go wrong, that the proper orientation to the world is an anxious concern for what can go wrong. I would thus make it very difficult for these patients to have a 'corrective emotional experience' with me.

Windy Dryden: You have talked about indications where you would not at the outset of therapy mention the prospect of a therapeutic impasse occurring. What would be some of the indications that might lead you to talk about this at the beginning of therapy?

Paul Wachtel: Well, one indication would be when I found myself having a sense of apprehension about the work. Another indication might be the person who forms a quick and total dependent attachment to someone. You gain a sense from their description of their history that these are people who constantly place all their eggs in one basket and are devastated when things don't work out. Although therapy requires that such a person make me an important person for him, I want to prevent myself from being boxed in later on by that. So when I raise, at the outset, that there may be many therapists who might be helpful to that person, I am doing so with a particular purpose in mind. I am attempting to forestall the situation that might occur later on where that person is so involved with me that I may have great difficulty raising the issue of lack of progress.

Indeed I do believe strongly that probably the ideal therapeutic endeavour would be a series of relatively short experiences with a number of different therapists. It is in the very nature of human relationships that only one facet of oneself can be revealed in relation to one single other person and therefore that only a portion of the potential change possible can occur in relation to one particular other. There is a kind of grandiosity that is often embodied in the attitudes of therapists that they can be all things to all people. It is very important that we begin to question this assumption. I also think that it is important that we help patients to question it as well. One way to do this is to communicate to patients—'Get what you can from me, I hope that it will be quite valuable, but it is not all you are going to get in life.'

Windy Dryden: Have you found that raising this issue with patients prone to become overly dependent has offset later negative effects with them?

Paul Wachtel: I think the best that I can say is that it helps to lay the groundwork. Unfortunately, we don't have magic bullets in psychotherapy. It would be nice if we did. One of the reasons that I like the title of your book so much is that doing therapy inevitably involves dilemmas. There is no way to avoid dilemmas. The best one can do is to mitigate them and help to make them constructive experiences. In a sense, psychotherapy is a kind of crisis. What we know about crises is that they can bring out the worst in people, but they can also be the opportunity for useful change. I think the dilemmas that occur in psychotherapy are similar. The pain, the difficulty and the conflict cannot be eliminated. It cannot be avoided. Certainly the formulations, cautions and verbalizations that I am talking about here are not sufficient. It is not as if I say something and then set the person straight.

That clearly is not the case. Rather I am trying to create a tone, an atmosphere in which I have got a better chance of having the total body of forces move in a positive rather than a negative direction.

Windy Dryden: Let's talk about a situation where this dilemma has really become acute. There you are, working with a patient, change hasn't occurred and yet you fear raising this issue may do harm. What kind of internal dialogue are you having at that time?

Paul Wachtel: One that includes an ethical dimension. I think that the therapy literature ought to address ethical issues a good deal more than it does. There are real questions about the nature of my conflicting responsibilities towards this person. On the one hand, I have the responsibility not to be hurtful and on the other hand as a therapist I am supposed to be honest and act responsibly. I am supposed to be non-exploitive. These are the conflicts within me that I start to wrestle with.

One of the things that my thoughts often turn to is how to word comments to patients. You can phrase the same message very differently by using different sets of words. Surprisingly little attention has been paid to this in the therapy literature. I have written a little about this[2] and so has Daniel Wile,[3] a very creative therapist on the West Coast. The question is, how can I communicate the basic situation to the person in a way that he is most likely to be able to hear it? Clearly euphemism alone is not going to be helpful. People see through euphemisms. They can be experienced as insulting. You don't want to say something positive when there isn't some emotional ballast behind it. On the other hand, the kind of direct confrontation that some therapists like to make can be brutal and insensitive. And I do think one needs to put things most of the time relatively gently. I say most of the time because there are also people who take gentleness as an insult and while one would want to raise that as an issue and not simply go along with it, one also wants to speak the patient's language.

Windy Dryden: As you mentioned earlier there are no magic bullets to guide your work. Have you had any cases where you have phrased this message gently, caringly and therapeutically and yet the patient still became extremely hurt, extremely depressed and deteriorated as a result?

Paul Wachtel: Well, fortunately I haven't had the experience of someone really deteriorating in the face of my raising the issue. I have certainly encountered a patient being distressed by it and what I have found useful is to say something like: 'We have a dilemma here together. Let's look at what goes on. If I suggest to you that we ought to stop, that feels to you like I am not interested, or I don't care about you, or you have failed and so on. And if I *don't* suggest we stop (or at least consider the possibility) you sense that we are both colluding in something that doesn't work for you. And somehow or other whichever way we approach it, it doesn't feel right for you. Let's see if we can look at that experience and find other things in your life that feel similar.' Usually when the situation becomes particularly intractable in this way, it is not a unique experience for the patient. It is representative of the patient's own life dilemmas and conflicts and sometimes it can be very useful for the patient to examine that. Raising it often allows me to continue to work productively. It is not, by any means, always the sign that you ought to be stopping. I think what is important is not so much that you persuade the patient to stop the work but that you persuade the patient to face that it has not been working well. Sometime this allows the two of you to work well together.

Windy Dryden: You mentioned the importance of wording in raising this issue with patients. Perhaps you can give more examples of how you would phrase your interventions.

Paul Wachtel: I think that one of the things that is important to consider here is the attributional nature of what one is discussing. Instead of presenting it as your decision as a therapist that this is not going well and your pronouncement that this ought to stop, it is better to encourage the patient to find a way to say something about it. And so my initial comments tend to be questions: 'How do you feel this is going?' 'Have you had any thoughts or questions or hesitancies about how we are doing?' If I make an interpretive statement it tends to be both interpretive and attributional at the same time. I might say to the person: 'I have the sense that you have been wondering if we are getting anywhere.' I will usually try to find some peg to hang that on, something that the person has communicated that has given me that sense. I will then say things like: 'You know, one of the things that we are up against is that you are sensing something isn't quite right for you. Something here is not going the way you hoped and yet there is something that seems very scary about saying that. There is something either about what it will mean about the success of the enterprise for you, or how I will take it—whether I will be able to stand it—that makes you feel that you can't address that. If you get nothing else out of this experience, then in a sense, if you can say to me: "You know I am not sure at this point in my life that this is the best thing for me". If you can say, "Maybe I can look elsewhere and get something else," I will feel that we have done something worthwhile and I think you can feel you have done something worthwhile.' I think with that sort of tone, one can begin to address some of these issues.

Windy Dryden: Returning to the dilemma, I can imagine that with someone who is really disturbed, where change isn't occurring and where you get a sense that if you raise this issue deterioration will occur, then you are faced with the situation where you are just working to stabilize this patient.

Paul Wachtel: Doing supportive therapy is usually not the most rewarding or stimulating kind of work for therapists. It is often boring, repetitive, unrewarding. And yet sometimes we clearly find ourselves in situations where it is our therapeutic obligation to put in a boring, unrewarding hour each week so that you can keep someone going in a fairly stabilized way, living a life that more or less works for them. It is not what you would have hoped for them but it is a lot better than what might be. Sometimes that is simply what we have to do. Therapeutic work cannot always be tremendously exiciting. Doing therapy is one of the most exciting, but also one of the most difficult and often either boring or frustrating or disturbing, kinds of work. I think we all have to be prepared for a certain balance amongst these experiences. So doing supportive, stabilizing therapy is the price we pay. The price becomes less when you can face that, and when you can recognize that for this person, at this time, it seems to be the best you can do. That helps to some extent.

Windy Dryden: Playing devil's advocate for a moment, I would imagine that some of your more traditionally analytic colleagues might say: 'Well, look, this therapist's sense of impatience is in itself a problem. Through his impatience, he is communicating subtle demands on the patient which the patient experiences and the impasse is caused by that.' How would you deal with this particular criticism?

Paul Wachtel: I am sure that sometimes this is true. It is in the nature of therapeutic work that every therapist is going to have certain characteristics that, some of the time, get in the way. I can imagine that my desire to see change manifestly can sometimes get in the way. On the other hand, I am suspicious of how readily therapists can be accused in the present psychoanalytic atmosphere of having excessive therapeutic zeal. It is a phrase one hears not infrequently. Freud, we are told, had relatively little therapeutic zeal. Sometimes, my zeal can be excessive but I think more often in the contemporary psychotherapeutic scene the problem tends to lie in the other direction. More often the problem is therapists who have insufficient therapeutic zeal. They are perfectly content to sit and collect their fees and be fascinated by what the person is saying and not worry about whether the patient is changing. It is easier on the therapist and may be easier on the patient. But in the long run, in most instances, I don't think it is in the patient's interest. I am sure that I don't find the correct balance in every single case. But I would rather err at least somewhat on the side of being an advocate for change, than err, as so often occurs, in the direction of disavowing any responsibility for change to occur.

Windy Dryden: Disavowing responsibility and therefore giving patients an excessive sense of responsibility?

Paul Wachtel: I do think that it can lead to the patient feeling an excessive sense of responsibility. But one of the things that also happens in therapy is that patients are often gratified by the therapeutic process and the patient himself does not notice that in the rest of his life nothing much has happened. I have frequently heard people whose lives are a mess talk about how wonderful their therapist is. And what they mean is that seeing the therapist is the only good hour in their week. Or the only good two, three or five hours in the week. That to me is not much of a testimonial to the therapist. I think that this is not uncommon. I think that how good the experience is in the moments you are together is not the best criterion. The criterion is how good is the person's life? Has the quality of that person's life improved or not?

Windy Dryden: You seem in that statement to have some reservations concerning the extent to which we should use a patient's self-report as an indication of therapeutic change.

Paul Wachtel: I do think we should take patients' self-reports very seriously in some ways. Ultimately most psychotherapy has subjective criteria. To be sure, there are times—for example, if you are working with a sex offender—when changes in external behaviour from a societal point of view are perhaps paramount. However, for most people seeking psychotherapy the single most important criteron is whether they really feel better in their daily lives. The old joke about the patient who says, 'I still have my symptoms but now I don't mind them,' in some ways is not as silly a notion as it sounds. We *are* dealing with subjective matters. The problem is that we all know that people can rationalize, people can and do deceive themselves, people can have a kind of veneer of words about something being better, and yet you can look at them and people know that they are not leading as full or as rich a life as they could. So I would want to take the patient's subjective report very seriously, but I would also want to take very seriously the experience of others around them.

One of the things that led, in an indirect way, to my quesitoning of the traditional analytic precepts that I was trained in was looking at my colleagues, all of whom had been through classical analysis of one sort or another. They had had what was in effect being portrayed as the Rolls-Royce of therapies, and yet my experience—and whenever I have mentioned this to colleagues nobody has contradicted this—when I began to look at the community of therapists around me was that I just did not see, by any means, a community of *Ubermenschen*. In fact I see a community which is, at best, average in mental health. And many would have reason to question even that statement. So the Rolls-Royce does not seem to produce people one envies. Although those therapists spoke highly of their analyses and said how important it was in their lives, I made my judgment of their experiences somewhat independent of their self-report. It did not appear as if they were leading as full or as rich a life as one would hope would be the case after such an experience.

Windy Dryden: You mentioned a word earlier which stands out for me, and that is the word 'veneer'. It seems as if we have been talking today about two kinds of 'veneer'. One which prompted you to question the efficacy of traditional psychoanalysis and psychoanalytic therapy, that is the 'veneer' of mental health of your colleagues. I think you have also brought into focus another 'veneer' where a patient may say things are fine, and yet you have reason to question that. I see a link between those two. I don't know if you do.

Paul Wachtel: Well. that is interesting. What you are talking about in the second meaning of veneer, I think of in terms of paradox—particularly the paradoxical effects of raising with people questions about their dissatisfactions about therapy. If one wants one's patients to praise the work you are doing the best way is to say: 'Gee I am wondering if we are getting anywhere.' All you have to do is do that and the patient will give lavish descriptions of how terrific it has been. I find that over and over again. It is ironic that if you allude to this, the people who seem to me to be getting the least from therapy are the one who most vociferously tell me how important I am in their life. Now, I think what's involved in this situation is part of what we were talking about before. These patients are being both protective of me and of themselves. There is something that feels very shaky to them and they have a real need to bolster this shakiness by presenting the therapy as going well. There is something that is very threatening about the idea that this parental-like relationship is not going well. It feels like a replication of some kind of perceived parental failure. This is very much at the heart of the dilemma. It is not just a personal dissatisfaction. It is not just disappointing someone. It is the spectre of another parental failure that is involved. The parental failure may be in part an imagined one. It is not necessarily that the parents did the wrong thing. But something went on while the person was being raised that did not work well for that person. That is very often the hardest thing of all for them to face. Even people who are very critical of their parents find it very hard to face this. It is very easy for someone to constantly moan and bitch about what their parents were like and yet at the same time be extremely protective towards their parents, which to some degree often comes out in their relationship with me. They need to make me the good parent.

Windy Dryden: For fear of hurting the parent?

Paul Wachtel: Fear of hurting the parent and also a fear of a kind of despair that can come if one really fully accepts the idea that the parent, who in some way or another always remains a kind of fantasized mediator of reality, can't do the job. I mean we all depend on mummy and daddy, somewhere in some deep recess of the mind.

Windy Dryden: You would also say, wouldn't you, that therapists have to face the related fear of not being able to do the job with particular patients?

Paul Wachtel: Yes, the task we take on is in some ways a terrifying one. To work with people who have a history of thwarting themselves and to think that we can reverse this trend. Inevitably at least part of the work involves our getting caught up in that pattern. There is a kind of quicksand involved here and therapy is the art of extricating oneself from quicksand; that's not the easiest thing to do.

NOTES

1. For a discussion of the 'corrective emotional experience' see: Alexander, F. and French, T. M. (1946) *Psychoanalytic Therapy: Principles and Application*, New York: Ronald Press.
2. See: Wachtel, P. (1980) What should we say to our patients? On the wording of therapists' comments. *Psychotherapy: Theory, Research and Practice*, 17(2), 183–188.
3. See for example: Wile, D. (1981) *Couple Therapy: A Nontraditional Approach*, New York: Wiley.

DISCUSSION ISSUES

1. *What dilemmas (if any) do you experience in continuing to see a client who does not seem to be improving? How have you attempted to resolve these dilemmas?*
2. *Do you share Paul Wachtel's contention that working with a client who gets worse during therapy is less discouraging than working with a client who remains unchanged? If so, why? If not, why not?*
3. *How prepared are you to discuss with clients, at the outset of therapy, the possibility that therapeutic impasses might occur? What factors determine your decisions in this matter?*
4. *How do you manage your own feelings when you dislike a client? How willing are you to voice such feelings in therapy? Under what conditions do you consider it to be appropriate (and inappropriate) for you to do so?*
5. *Do you think that clients are better served by having brief periods of therapy with different therapists or an extended period with a single therapist?*
6. *To what extent do you base your self-esteem on your therapeutic results?*

CHAPTER FOURTEEN

Missing Links and Lacunae

An interview with Arnold Lazarus

In 1972, after spending two years at Yale University as the director of clinical training in the psychology department, Arnold Lazarus joined Rutgers University in New Brunswick, New Jersey, as a professor II. This rank is reserved for those full professors who have achieved scholarly eminence in their fields of inquiry, and he was sufficiently flattered by this offer to give up his post at a prestigious Ivy League institution. He has not regretted this move. In 1974, Rutgers was one of the pioneers of a new movement in clinical psychology—the development of a doctor of psychology degree (PsyD) intended for those clinicians who were primarily interested in practice rather than research. Thus, Arnold Lazarus moved to the Graduate School of Applied and Professional Psychology (he had been the chairperson of the department of psychology at Rutgers University College) and has been primarily a 'therapist trainer' over the past decade. He also has a private practice in Princeton, New Jersey, and serves as a consultant to several state agencies, private and public.

Arnold is a fellow of several professional associations, and a diplomate of two professional boards, and in 1982 he was elected into the newly formed National Academy of Practice in Psychology. He has received several other professional honours and awards and is listed in Who's Who in America *and in* Who's Who in the World. *He has authored, co-authored or edited ten books and presently serves on the editorial boards of eleven journals. He has published over 120 articles and has lectured extensively throughout America as well as in overseas countries, including England, Norway, Sweden, Israel and South Africa. His main achievement has been to develop an approach and therapy known as Multimodal therapy which is gaining professional recognition throughout America and abroad.*

Arnold's major interests focus on the treatment of marriage problems, sex problems, stress-related difficulties, and various phobias. For many years he has been aware of the pernicious effects that arise when therapists are wedded to specific theories, and he has advocated a technically eclectic stance. He still ponders an essential dichotomy—those who subscribe to measurement, observation and objectivism, versus the champions of intuition, holism and subjectivism—and is interested in a type of integration that would not end up as a mishmash of incompatible ideas. He considers that we are very much in need of better aetiological and antecedent factors than our present theories tend to yield. In other words, he feels that every approach to psychological theory and therapy is weak on basic issues of causality. This is perhaps the most significant gap in the clinical arena. As Arnold says: 'Often we do not know "What makes Johnny run", or why he bothers to move at all!' These sorts of lacunae are explored in the following interview.

Windy Dryden: Would you like to state your therapeutic dilemma in your own words?

Arnold Lazarus: The first dilemma concerns why some people exhibit levels of disturbance for no 'good' reason. In other words, one's thorough investigation fails to pinpoint antecedent factors that adequately explain the individual's ongoing problems. It is always possible to talk in broad terms about a genetic diathesis, about the impact of various stressors and conflicts, but these vague, nebulous terms don't crystalize what is really happening in the individual cases. Consequently, the therapist remains perplexed as to why these people are so unhappy, and why they are functioning so poorly. This would characterize approximately 5 per cent of my patients at present.

I am thinking in particular of a young, 35 year-old physician who suffers from panic, general claustrophobia and pervasive anxiety. He experiences a variety of phobias such as bridge phobia, claustrophobia and acrophobia. He avoids crowds and is generally incapacitated by these symptoms. Although he is a very successful internist, life for him is an uphill battle because of these symptoms. While searching for antecedent factors, I found that his problems seemed to start at the time when he was in medical school, under a lot of stress, shortly after the demise of his grandmother of whom he was very fond. However, these vague and general precipitants don't hang together. They do not account for the fact that this person today is as disturbed as he is. And, my therapeutic attempts to remedy his disturbances have followed the usual gamut of therapies from relaxation, bio-feedback, and special breathing exercises, to various desensitization methods, you name it, without any significant therapeutic impact. I might mention that before seeing me, he had seen a number of traditional therapists, and their brand of insight seemed to be as accurate as pre-Columbian maps and of as much benefit as those maps would be to a present-day navigator. But I can claim no better results with my broad spectrum of Multimodal methods because I think, very largely, I have failed to identify the true antecedents and maintaining factors. To call him a Type A personality, since he is rather pressured and harried, is true, and to some extent, by teaching him slowing-down tactics, he has improved in that regard, but the dilemma is that we have been unable to account for his pathology.

A similar case in point is a 39 year-old woman whom I have seen on and off for the past ten years who has also been to numerous other therapists. In fact, her dossier reads like a 'Who's Who' in psychotherapy. She complains of intermittent depressions that don't seem to be typically uni-polar or bi-polar and don't fit into any of the relevant DSM III[1] categories. She complains of a wide range of psychosomatic disorders and has seen numerous physicians. Indeed she recently lost her uterus to one of them. Again if one looks at her family history, at her developmental stages and phases, one can point to nothing in her life that truly accounts for the extent of her incapacities. She suffers from extreme facial pain which is a tension bi-product, and bio-feedback, relaxation, self-hypnosis, have done nothing for her. The only thing that seems to help is Valium or other tranquillizers which she has not abused but seems to take almost as a placebo, because she takes very small doses. Once more this is a dilemma, because in trying to understand what this is all about and what one can do to remedy matters, all therapists, myself included, have drawn a blank. So those are some instances of the dilemma of failing to identify the antecedents of ongoing problems and who or what is maintaining them.

Windy Dryden: Looking at this a little more closely, it seems as if understanding the antecedents and the maintaining factors are very important in helping you to choose a range of appropriate therapeutic strategies and therapeutic techniques to implement these strategies. Is that correct?

Arnold Lazarus: It is important for me to feel that I am selecting my procedures based upon a properly formulated assessment of the case. However, there have been other cases where I have not been able to pinpoint these factors, but have used a mélange of well-established techniques and the people have benefitted. Again it is a dilemma in the sense that these people will then exit from therapy as smiling, satisfied customers and I, the therapist, remain perplexed as to what it was that produced the salubrious result. As a *clinician*, that does not bother me as long as the people get well and stay well. However, as a *researcher*, I would like to try and put my finger on the processes that were operative. So it is a problem, and it is not a problem, at one and the same time.

Windy Dryden: So, as you were saying, when you don't quite understand the antecedents and the maintaining factors of the patient's problems and the patients get better, that does not present too much of a problem for you. You would like to understand, but the fact that they have been helped is the main concern for you. But it sounds as if, when you don't understand, and your range of therapeutic techniques and strategies don't work then the dilemma becomes more acute.

Arnold Lazarus: That is perfectly right.

Windy Dryden: What attempts have you made to resolve this dilemma?

Arnold Lazarus: The attempts to resolve this dilemma have been threefold. First, discussion with colleagues, either by having them sit in on some of these difficult cases, or by having them hear my outline and give advice, suggestions and input. Second, I have searched through the literature for answers that might be published in tomes hitherto neglected. Third, I have often invented new procedures in the hope that somehow these would produce a result where everything else had failed. I am referring to the person who keeps coming for therapy and apparently does do what one asks them to do. They are not the resistant cases (we can get to those next as dilemma number two), but are cooperative people who are doing what the state of the art suggests they should be doing and yet derive no benefit.

Windy Dryden: In accounting for this phenomenon it would be possible to say: 'Well, the state of the art is still in a pretty primitive stage and perhaps we would be able to help these people twenty or thirty years down the line because we would perhaps have invented or developed very powerful therapeutic methods and techniques.' Another way of explaining it would be to say: 'Well, look. There may be some people who do not respond to therapeutic endeavours. Full stop.'

Arnold Lazarus: My guess is that we are exceedingly weak on aetiology and I am referring to all theories. In this respect there are some theories such as Freudian theory, or Eysenckian theory, that point to clear-cut antecedents. If you are an Eysenckian there is no doubt whatsoever that the problem is one of Type B Pavlovian conditioning which is notoriously resistant to extinction—there is your fatuous answer! The analyst will of course talk about fixations, unconscious conflicts and putative repressions. They have these immediate answers which just do not help the practising clinician to devise appropriate strategies and tactics to offset these people's problems. Now I am not even referring to certain people who seem beyond the pale — the ones that just cannot be helped. Nor am I referring to florid psychotics, or sociopathic personalities, or addictive-substance abusers. I am not even referring to that genre of pathology which most clinicians would shy away from. I am just talking about your common-or-garden-variety neurotic who *should* by all that we know, be responsive to our ministrations, but nevertheless does not respond. Whether it is appropriate to say that they just have to be put into an unhelpable group, or whether it is that we don't yet know how to pinpoint the antecedent and maintaining factors, remains perplexing. I put my money on the latter. I feel that we need to develop more accurate assessment procedures that will enable us to pinpoint genuine developmental processes, more effectively identify basic problems, and ultimately provide solutions thereto.

Windy Dryden: Do you have any idea what these new assessment procedures might look like?

Arnold Lazarus: My guess is that they would be multi-dimensional. They would help us to ferret out some elusive interactions, some, for example, cognitive-imagery processes that are very difficult to identify at present, or some kind of subtle firing order of the different personality dimensions that trigger subtle affective reactions. I have in mind a situation where clinicians will be helped to identify a pivotal sequence that can be interrupted at a crucial point and make a world of difference to the patient. Something along those lines. I am vague because this is truly a dilemma for me.

Windy Dryden: Your hunch is that where you are successful with those problems wherein the aetiology and maintaining factors are vague, you somehow manage fortuitously to actually hit on this vaguely understood firing order by using your complex range of therapeutic techniques.

Arnold Lazarus: It has very often been referred to as the 'fishnet approach'—you toss in the net and if you are lucky you get a rich yield. And sometimes the best you can do clinically is to toss in the net. This means when utilizing a barrage of techniques, as luck would have it, you happen to hit on some correct sequencing, or some correct ordering, and, *voilà*, there is a change. Again, as a *clinician* that is fine, but as a *scientist* that is not good enough, and it does remain perplexing.

Windy Dryden: And then if you could find some previously elusive factor then some therapeutic strategy would suggest itself?

Arnold Lazarus: Yes, most likely.

Windy Dryden: Does that necessarily follow?

Arnold Lazarus: Well, at least something could be invented to fit the sequence. I say that because ever since developing the concept of 'tracking' and 'modality firing orders' I have found that hitherto unreachable cases are more likely to fall into place and respond. A typical case in point is the individual who says, 'I have these attacks of anxiety out of the blue, for no apparent reason,' then you go through a tracking procedure with the client who discovers that these things do not come out of the blue. A given case may begin with a sensory reaction, followed by an image, followed by a cognition, followed by an affective reaction, followed by a behaviour. When you are able to pinpoint a particular sequence you can then help the person overcome it by prescribing therapies that fit that firing order. I became impressed by the fact that people with identical symptomatology can have very different firing orders and therefore need different orders of therapy or types of therapy. That discovery really advanced my clinical effectiveness. It is this sort of thing that I am referring to. Something like this taken a step further might elucidate some of these problems we are addressing.

Windy Dryden: Another viewpoint is that your Multimodal perspective may be getting in the way of determining what may be hindering therapeutic progress.

Arnold Lazarus: I know what you are getting at. Of course, every therapist is limited by his or her conceptual framework, by his or her implicit or explicit theories. Clearly, we all do in therapy what makes personal sense to us. We all have at the very least an implicit idea of why people develop emotional and behavioural problems, and this will affect what we do and don't do in therapy, and in this way our conceptual frameworks could be getting in the way. The Multimodal framework, as you know, is very broad and flexible and is by no means monolithic. There are so many different options that the structure, *per se*, is probably less likely to get in the way. However, what I have done with a lot of these cases to which I am referring is sent them to clinicians whose views are quite divergent from my own, on the assumption that they would have something to offer these poor people who have not responded to my ministrations. So I have referred people to bio-energetic analysts in the Philadelphia and New York areas who are reputed to be experts. I have sent people for EST training.[2] I have sent people for Rolfing.[3] I have sent people to almost occult individuals who are well outside of my conceptual framework, to determine whether or not help may be forthcoming. Occasionally that has worked. I think that people enter therapy with certain expectations and this might be at the core of what we are talking about. If the clients' expectations are not met, if what the therapist is doing is at variance with what the client thinks the therapist should be doing, positive results are unlikely to ensue.

I must say, however, that referral to esoteric practitioners has not been the rule; it is by far the exception. Moreover, referral to people well outside the Multimodal framework is not done capriciously; it is done when I sense that maybe there is something there which may be of benefit to a particular individual. And, indeed, if this worked consistently I would feel a lot more confident and it wouldn't be a dilemma because then I could say: 'Well, whenever I am unable to formulate the antecedents and maintaining factors it means that this person will probably be helped by a practitioner of an occult school using ESP.' Thus, it would not be a dilemma because I would know what to do. It remains a dilemma because in most cases, even when I have stepped right outside of my framework, there did not seem to be much benefit. The case I referred to, i.e. the 39 year-old woman, has seen a veritable army of therapists both competent and incompetent, respectable and well within the lunatic fringe. Over ten years, the impact is almost zero, which is the strange and perplexing thing. Too many people tend to explain away such cases by invoking 'resistance' or even by platitudes such as, 'She doesn't want to get better.'

Windy Dryden: Taking an argument that you probably are familiar with, what would happen to this woman if she did get over her problems? I have the notion of a woman who has been given fabulous attention from esteemed practitioners. You know the argument.

Arnold Lazarus: I have never been impressed with that argument because I don't think that the benefits outweigh the liabilities. She is in too much discomfort to be compensated adequately by the stimulating company of professionals.

Windy Dryden: Even charming ones like yourself!

Arnold Lazarus: Even the most charming of all. That doesn't mean me!

Windy Dryden: So having entertained the notion of searching for an explanation outside your framework it led you back to your original hypothesis, namely that there is some effect there but it is so subtle that it escapes our ability to detect and assess it.

Arnold Lazarus: My notion is there is an answer if only we can find it. It exists.

Windy Dryden: Then it will remain a dilemma until assessment procedures have been developed with the power to tease out these effects.

Arnold Lazarus: Not only assessment procedures but indeed a general step forward in our understanding of human beings, in general psychological knowledge. I feel that we have at the moment so many competing theories that nobody truly understands human functioning and behaviour. I think that we have got the age-old example of the committee who has put together some hybrid that doesn't quite fit the animal that they intended to construct, or the blind people feeling parts of an elephant and imagining what the total animal looks like. I think this is where we are in our field at the moment. We don't have a true integrated picture of human functioning.

We have got little sketches here and there. A kind of mosaic that has not been put together.

Windy Dryden: And such advances in assessment that you are seeking may be linked with advances in our understanding of human beings and how they develop, etc. Would that be correct?

Arnold Lazarus: Yes, that is correct. You know, I feel that the reason that this dilemma persists is because of the rival factions that exist in the field. Some time ago I wrote: 'I am opposed to the advancement of psychoanalysis, to the advancement of Gestalt therapy, to the advancement of existential therapy, to the advancement of behavior therapy or to the advancement of any delimited school of thought. I would like to see an advancement in psychological knowledge, an advancement in the understanding of human interaction in the alleviation of suffering and in the know-how of therapeutic intervention' (Lazarus, 1977, p. 553[4]).

And this is what I am getting at when I say that we don't have that global integrated understanding at this stage. Instead we have pockets of wisdom, islands of information in an ocean of ignorance.

Windy Dryden: And I guess, until that ocean begins to be explored a little bit more, some of these patients will continue to have a tough time swimming in their troubled waters.

Arnold Lazarus: Yes. That is well put.

Windy Dryden: Shall we go on to the second dilemma?

Arnold Lazarus: The second dilemma is the ubiquitous problem that has sometimes been called 'resistance'. The term is unfortunate, and I have a chapter with Allen Fay in Wachtel's (1982)[5] book decrying the concept and denouncing it in some ways, but also trying to explicate what it is all about. Here is an example. Typically, one gives homework assignments to clients, and when they fail to do their homework they are called 'unco-operative' or 'resistant'. Sometimes this is because the therapist has not ensured that the client truly appreciates the value of homework exercises. The client does not understand the rationale, so does not do the exercise. Sometimes the client is just not in favour of self-help in any way, shape or form, and will simply not cooperate. At other times the specific homework assignments are perceived by the client as irrelevant to his or her problems. On other occasions, the homework is not seen as cost-effective, i.e. it is either too difficult to carry out or too time-consuming or both. And sometimes the assigned tasks are just too threatening. But let us assume that a clinician, well versed in these procedures, has determined that none of the foregoing applies and the client comes back without having done his or her homework, evincing no change. This becomes a dilemma.

I want to give you a case in point. A man in his mid-thirties, with a somewhat Calvinistic religious upbringing, found that upon getting married, he had zero sex with his first wife—who divorced him for that reason. Prior to marriage, he was very active sexually with other women and with his wife premaritally. But the moment they married all sexual activity ceased. When asked for an explanation, he said that he thinks it has something to do with a misconception (he so labelled it), namely that respectable people do not engage in the frenetic activity called sexual intercourse. He added that when you have made a woman respectable by marrying her, she is now 'a wife' and that this is not the kind of thing that a respectable man and woman do in their bedroom, living room or anywhere else. (I think Freud called this the 'Madonna Complex'.) When the wife divorced him, he resumed a very active sex life and met his second wife where the same pattern was enacted. This time there is a child almost a year old. And, once more, the patient articulates the stupidity and ridiculousness of his Calvinistic thoughts (that as a pillar of the community, as a respectable husband and father, and a respectable married couple, sex is off-limits, except perhaps for procreation). He says he loves his wife. His wife supports the fact he is kind, loving, attentive and caring in all respects, but not with regard to sexual participation. He is aware of the fact that he stands a good chance of ruining his second marriage and breaking up the family. He in fact had spoken of having a second child. His wife rather facetiously asked how the child would be born!

Again, prior to seeing me, this man saw a very experienced behaviour therapist who put him through a most elaborate desensitization procedure on the assumption that there was some anxiety associated with sexual participation and performance. I have done an elaborate amount of cognitive disputation, cognitive restructuring, even introduced a variety of threat-inducing reactions. I called in a priest to give him a talking-to, and the net result has been zero movement. By the way, I asked him what would happen if his beloved son were kidnapped, and he were told by the kidnappers that unless for the next month he had intercourse with his wife three times a week, his child would be put to death, but if he succeeded in having inter-course three times a week, his child would then be returned unharmed. How positive was he that he could get his child back unharmed? He answered 'absolutely positive'. I pointed out to him that when a metaphori-cal gun is pointed to his head, he is willing to perform, but not in order to save his marriage. Moreover, his wife is not the kind of demanding female who insists on complete sexual intercourse, but says that she would be quite satisfied if he were loving, kissing, caressing, fondling, and perhaps brought her to orgasm a few times a week with manual or oral stimulation. Masters and Johnson have stressed that no man can will an erection, so I thought there might be a performance anxiety at the base of his problem. Not so. It remains a perplexing dilemma as to why this man who apparently dearly loves his wife, and wants to preserve the marriage, will not do what is necessary. I asked him whether if his wife suffered from an affliction that required a fifteen-minute massage of her back three times a week he would do it, and he said absolutely. Well, why then would he not massage her clitoris three times a week? A most perplexing dilemma.

Windy Dryden: Now, you mention this second dilemma in terms of understanding the determinants of the problem as opposed to the first dilemma where the determinants of the problem were only vaguely understood. Here you are sure that you understand the determinants . . . and he actually desires a change in the stated direction, but that no therapeutic procedures can be brought to bear on this problem. Is this correct?

Arnold Lazarus: Not entirely. There is an overlap with the first dilemma in that I don't feel that I am fully on top of this case. The difference is that I can point to what appears to be logical determinants—his Calvinistic upbring-ing, his very poor relationship with his mother, and various other factors that seem to have a bearing. One of the analysts he had seen thought that this was an unconscious hostility to women, generalizing from mother to all other females. Again, that kind of reasoning seems rather strained. There is nothing else in his behaviour to suggest there is an underlying hostility. Nevertheless, I have failed to identify an elusive fulcrum and lever that would get this case moving. The difference, however, is that at least I can pinpoint some apparently meaningful antecedents. The dilemma in this case focusses on what it is that prevents an intelligent, apparently highly motivated man from performing a 'task' that would ensure his marriage happiness and a successful future as a family man, which, as far as I can see, he wishes to achieve. Now it is very easy for people to argue that the truth is that at some deep unconscious level there is a self-destructive tendency, that he wishes to punish himself, that he is besieged by such guilt that he doesn't feel himself worthy of happiness, and therefore the finest way to sabotage it is through this insidious, you might call it, marital suicide pact that he has entered into. That is perhaps like saying that the ultimate truth is that God in heaven is alive and well, and decided to issue a punishment for sins that his grandfather ten times removed had carried out several hundred years ago. Both of those kinds of explanations are equally fatuous because what can you do with them? So I come back to saying that that line of reasoning is counterproductive and I am left believing that he would like the happiness to which he feels he is entitled, and there is a basic lacuna. There is indeed, the more I think about it, an overlap between these two dilemmas, because presumably if the therapist is fully cognizant of all the factors, he or she will not find resistant clients because of knowing just how to proceed through the jungle. So these two are closely linked. Oh for a psychic compass!

Windy Dryden: You seem to be stating that what is common to both these dilemmas is that resistance in therapy occurs out of therapist ignorance, where the therapist is not able to adequately pinpoint subtle maintaining mechanisms.

Arnold Lazarus: Correct. That applies in most instances.

Windy Dryden: And once we pinpoint and understand them and develop established or new therapeutic techniques then resistance will not occur.

Arnold Lazarus: I think it is true that at least 90 per cent of resistance is due to therapist ignorance.

NOTES

1. The third edition of *Diagnostic and Statistical Manual of Mental Disorders*, the psychiatric classification system developed by the American Psychiatric Association.
2. Erhard Seminars Training: 'a brief but intense large-group experience the object of which is to get in touch with one's responsibility of one's being. Means

to this end include physical privation, guided meditation and confrontations and indoctrination by the group trainer.' (Kovel, J. (1978) *A Complete Guide to Therapy,* Brighton: Harvester Press, p. 262).

3. Rolfing: 'a method of firm and vigorous touch to release feelings bound up with deep musculature'. (Liss, J. (1974) *Free to Feel,* London: Wildwood House, p. 12).

4. Lazarus, A. A. (1977) Has behaviour therapy outlived its usefulness? *American Psychologist,* 32(7), 500–554.

5. Wachtel, P. L. (Ed) (1982) *Resistance: Psychodynamic and Behavioral Approaches,* New York: Plenum.

DISCUSSION ISSUES

1. *How important is it for you to understand the antecedent and maintaining factors of your client's problems in the practice of psychotherapy?*

2. *When clients do not improve as a result of therapy, what range of explanations do you employ in attempting to determine the reason(s) for the non-improvement?*

3. *Do you agree with Arnold Lazarus that 90 per cent of client resistance is due to therapist ignorance?*

4. *How do you cope with your own level of ignorance as a therapist?*

5. *How easy do you find it to refer clients to fellow professionals when therapeutic impasses are not resolved?*

CHAPTER FIFTEEN

The Psychotic Disguise

An interview with Don Bannister

Don Bannister is a member of the Medical Research Council external scientific staff and is based at the High Royds Hospital in West Yorkshire. He is engaged in a long-term research project applying personal construct theory (as originally proposed by George Kelly) to aspects of psychological disturbance. This has recently involved him in a study of the way in which patients newly admitted to psychiatric hospitals see their own problems, their underlying theory about their disorder and the interaction between their self-diagnosis and the hospital's official view. Currently he is involved in an investigation of the way in which children learn to construe themselves (to develop a picture of self) and ways in which this development may become problematic and lead to psychological distress.

As part of his general work on developing applications of personal construct theory Don has authored a number of books on the subject including Inquiring Man *with Fay Fransella (Penguin, 1980) and* The Evaluation of Personal Constructs *with Miller Mair (Academic Press, 1968).*

Much of Don's work stems from earlier studies he conducted at Bexley Hospital in Kent from 1960 to 1976, centring on the problem of schizophrenic thought disorder. In the course of this work he developed a test of thought disorder and undertook long term psychotherapy with many so-called schizophrenics. His account of the dilemma that follows stems from this experience gained in working with long-stay psychiatric patients.

Windy Dryden: OK, Don, would you like to put your dilemma in your own words?

167

Don Bannister: Let me put the dilemma in context first. A lot of my work in the field of psychotherapy has been done with clients categorized as psychotic and nine times out of ten they were long-stay patients in a psychiatric hospital. The dilemma that I am going to talk about has not been frequently discussed in psychotherapy circles because there is a kind of superstition that psychotics are unsuitable for psychotherapy. I have always been puzzled by this. In its extreme form, this view states that the only people who are suitable for therapy are young, relatively educated, intelligent, relatively articulate and able to form warm relationships. In other words they are in better shape than I am; so I can never understand why they need therapy. Even people who take a wider perspective than that would still say that you cannot do productive therapy with psychotics. Now I believe that you can carry out useful psychotherapy with psychotics but it does have its own particular problems. The particular one that I want to talk about is the problem of how best psychotherapists can respond to delusional talk or delusional beliefs. By this I mean that the client will talk at length in a manner which is extremely puzzling and extremely difficult to relate to, in the sense that he is claiming things which you cannot accept as true. What I am referring to is similar to the layman's idea of madness. A man thinks he is Napoleon, Jesus Christ or a teapot, for example. Or he sees some complicated plot against him which is initiated by creatures from outer space. This is a kind of talk which the client is not going to filter out for the purposes of therapy since it is part of their way of communicating. Herein lies the dilemma: how to respond? There are a number of ways of responding to delusional talk which I and others have tried. They are tempting ways but I don't think they get anywhere. They certainly never get the client anywhere.

One classic way of responding is to *humour* the patient. This is commonly employed by nurses on wards. In humouring you pretend to agree that the client does have, for example, magical powers in his fingertips or that he is being persecuted by the Russians. You go along, you pretend to agree, you smile and say 'Yes' and you say 'How dreadful!' However this approach does not tackle the issue at all. It is a way of getting along with the client but you can't do psychotherapy that way. If your aim is to just keep the institution pleasant and orderly then it is all right but otherwise it's useless. In addition, I think, in the long run, it is quite dangerous for the client because it leaves him without landmarks. Try and imagine yourself in a situation where you say that something is black, and everybody says: 'Yes, you are absolutely right, it is black.' Then you change your mind, or even run a little test and say: 'No, it's white, definitely white.' Everybody then says: 'Yes, I see what you mean, it is white.' So the landmarks keep shifting. If everything you say is going to be agreed with, you have no way of finding out whether particular points of view make any more sense to people than others. You get lost in the flow of your own thoughts because people simply go along with whatever you say. I am sure that this in fact adds to the problems of the so-called psychotic, particularly at the stage when he or she is trying to do some reality testing. However, it is a very tempting response.

Another way out of the dilemma is to respond with *'rational argument'*. Instead of humouring the patient when he is saying these very odd and bizarre things, you argue the rational case. You say that you do not believe what the person is saying or that you find it hard to believe and you call for evidence or you put forward contrary ideas about it. This approach is quite tempting for the liberal rational psychotherapist. It not only seems the sensible thing to do—not to put up with this nonsense—but also it seems that you are doing a kindness by arguing with the patient. I think there are a number of difficulties about this approach. The first is that if you try it, and I have tried it—most people do at one time or another—you discover that the client is not only saying things you find it hard to believe but also they have different notions of evidence and a different kind of logical assessment of evidence from you. In other words, it is not just that their belief is odd, their way of arriving at that belief or defending it is odd. As a result you get into a familiar pattern. For example, the classic paranoid belief is impossible to refute, because it is most often based on a conspiracy theory. The person claims that his body is being shrivelled away by rays which are sent by Russian agents. Suppose he makes a claim that is apparently checkable—he locates the source of the rays in a particular building. If you take the person across and demonstrate that there is no machinery in that building then this is because the agents have discovered that he knew about it and have transferred it to another building. Similarly if you get a lot of people to report that they don't agree with him, then obviously these people are in the pay of the Russian agents. In short, once you build up the notion of conspiracy there is no ultimate source of validation or invalidation. Everything could be seen to be a further layer in the conspiracy.

Windy Dryden: These are two attempts to solve the dilemma of how to respond to such talk that you have actually tried at some points in your career?

Don Bannister: Yes. I tried them in a rather desperate sort of way, not because either of them seemed likely to work but because . . . it is very hard to just ignore such talk.

Windy Dryden: Did you try to ignore it?

Don Bannister: That was my third approach, particularly with some very chronic patients. *Ignoring* such talk now seems to me to be similar to working on a token economy basis. When they said something that made sense I responded to it and when they said something that didn't make sense or was bizarre I just didn't respond to it. I would wait until they said something sensible and respond to that. Frankly, I didn't notice that it made any great difference. For a start it didn't resolve the problem of the many patients who brought their so-called delusions into almost everything that they said. It is thus very hard to find anything to respond to because everything they said contained delusional elements. This tack probably does no harm but it tends to leave you at square one.

The problem with all these three approaches is that you are left with a feeling of going around in circles. My experience was that I was not actually engaging the client. It is as if the client is talking to you pretty much as they would talk to anybody. So I didn't feel that I was establishing any particularly powerful relationship with them and again nothing much seemed to change in their behaviour or their distress.

Windy Dryden: Did you try these solutions in any particular order when you first started working with patients?

Don Bannister: Yes. I think there was a very definite order. In the very early days I think I tried a sort of mixture of humouring and ignoring but mainly humouring. I picked that up partly because it is in the culture, it is a cultural tradition which says don't argue with madmen, they may take an axe and chop your head off; be nice to madmen whatever you do. I think I went into hospitals with that in mind. The first time I worked in a psychiatric hospital was as a nursing assistant, and as a nurse you were quite definitely told by your charge nurse that you don't argue, you just go along with them; whatever they say you agree with and they will be fine. So I think that was my first strategy.

The rational argument approach came a lot later and was a bit more thought out. I tried to take a bit of Ellis's rational psychotherapy and apply it in working with so-called chronic psychotics by employing forceful and vigorous arguments. I actually followed that through systematically by trying to set up tests. For example, I would say to patients who claimed that they could tell what I was thinking: 'All right, I am going to think of the name of a town and I am going to write it down and put it in an envelope. You write down what I have written down.' So we set up a little telepathy experiment. However, it wouldn't work—they wouldn't guess the town but the interesting thing is that they would set up a special explanation for that. For instance they would get angry and say I had thought of the town that they had written down but that I had deliberately tricked them by writing down another town. Or there were particular reasons why the vibrations were not working on that day. I pushed it as far as actually trying to set up a whole series of tests. It was not that it produces no effect but the effects didn't seem terribly useful. Sometimes they responded with a fair degree of anger. It is not true to say that the person was unaffected by the argument or by the demonstrations. My guess is that they did feel their beliefs were a bit threatened but this didn't lead them to explore the beliefs or to question them. It was as if Kellyan 'hostility' took over. They attempted to extort validational evidence. They dug in more fiercely. There was a bit in the traditional psychiatric definition of delusions which says that a delusional belief is one which is unaffected by contrary evidence. Now I don't think that is true. I think the person who holds it is affected by contrary evidence but I think the effect is most often to get them further entrenched in their beliefs.

Windy Dryden: So where did that leave you?

Don Bannister: Well, that left me with the ignoring idea. One of the reasons for abandoning 'ignoring', incidentally, was that it creates a very artificial relationship which will not necessarily hold good. For instance, with one or two patients I ignored their delusional talk but worked with them in other ways. In a number of cases they left the hospital after many years and were apparently doing very well. However, in two cases that I clearly remember they were back within a matter of two or three months. When I explored what had happened to them and went to talk to their landladies and people they had worked with and so on, one of the big problems turned out to be that their workmates and others couldn't stand this funny bizarre talk and had either ostracized them or shouted at them. Or their landlady turned them out because she found she couldn't stand somebody talking about Russian spies and so on.

Windy Dryden: So, would it be true to say that your ignoring approach in fact didn't put them under any stress; however their workmates and other people wouldn't tolerate their talk and this proved too stressful for them?

Don Bannister: Yes, in other words you are not preparing them for the real world. Because in the real world people are going to be upset. People do get very upset by claims that you are Genghis Khan or whatever. So you are not doing them any favour by ignoring such talk in the therapy sessions.

Windy Dryden: So, you have mentioned three particular stances, all of which weren't particularly successful. Did you solve your dilemma at all by finding a stance that was more effective with these patients?

Don Bannister: Yes, I found one which made sense to me. I was able to apply it, get more response from using it and be more effective as a therapist with it.

Windy Dryden: What was that approach?

Don Bannister: I am trying to think of a phrase for it. The simplest way of putting it is to say that what I did was to start dealing with the theme of the delusion without dealing with its content. Part of this idea came from my increasing attempts to apply personal construct theory to my therapeutic work. A distinction that is made in this theory is between superordinate and subordinate constructions: what are the major underlying concerns as distinct from what you might call the immediate elements in what people are offering you? If I can give you an example. The first time I managed to stay with this approach and work it out, relatively successfully, was with a lad who employed a lot of delusional talk about conspiracies by the doctors in the hospital to assassinate him. He was talking, on one occasion that I can remember, about the 'fact' that the doctors had gotten together and were paying large sums of money to lorry drivers—who brought lorries into the grounds under the guise of bringing in goods—to try and run him down or squash him against the wall. They would be stationary until they saw him coming across the drive and then they would suddenly lunge at him. He was able to elaborate on this and talked about how much these lorry drivers were being paid and who was head of the ring that was doing it and so on. What I did was to take up the theme of the relationship between him and the doctors. I took it that he was asserting that the doctors disliked him intensely, that they did not care about his welfare, and that they would be quite happy if he came to no good end. In other words I extracted that as a *theme* and I talked about that theme with him. I asked questions about which particular doctors he felt disliked him, when had he thought they started disliking him, had he ever found any way of appealing to them and so on. I deliberately left aside the issue of the lorry drivers, the lurking round corners, and the crushing against walls. Instead I engaged very strongly with him on the issue of how he was regarded by the doctors in the hospital, particularly his feeling that he was regarded by them as disposable rubbish. This worked very well. The interesting thing was that he talked more and more about this theme and less and less about the lorry drivers. In fact, he had a case. He was a disliked patient. He was regarded as a chronic troublemaker who had been in hospital for many years and who had what was regarded as a hostile attitude. We talked further about whether this view extended to the nurses and to the other patients.

Another way of putting this would be to view his talk as a kind of unsignalled metaphor. If this material had been signalled as a metaphor we wouldn't have been in the least alarmed. If somebody said to you, 'I sometimes feel the doctors here hate me so much it wouldn't surprise me if they would like to see me run over by a lorry,' we might think of it as a rather colourful metaphor or figure of speech but we would respond in terms of the theme, of the doctors' dislike and so on. I am not sure that it explains anything to call such talk unsignalled metaphors because it leaves open the question of why the metaphors are not signalled.

Windy Dryden: You mention that one of your previous strategies was ignoring the person's delusional talk but that this did not involve putting anything in its place. Would it be true to say that searching for the central theme was in fact ignoring the delusional aspects but actually having something to target in its place.

Don Bannister: Yes, although the something must come *from* the 'delusions'. You mustn't just pick a subject and talk about it. You must actually be listening to the superordinate construction that underlies the delusion. All delusions have an assertion in them which can be abstracted, which in itself is not unreasonable. The only 'unreasonable' things are the concrete elaborations of the delusion.

Windy Dryden: Right. And these are the aspects that you ignore?

Don Bannister: Yes. I ignore them in the sense that I don't argue with them, I don't dispute them; what I do is to pay attention to the theme and work at length with the client at that superordinate level, whatever I think the theme is.

Windy Dryden: You use the concrete elaborations to help you identify the theme?

Don Bannister: Bearing in mind of course that I may initially guess wrong. However with luck I will realize that I am wrong and then I can guess again.

Windy Dryden: Was your interest in personal construct theory the major guiding principle in helping you to develop this approach?

Don Bannister: I think it was, except that even before I came across construct theory I had, like many people, an interest in what you might call consistent themes in people's lives, themes which are continuous and which have an essence over and above the particular context in which they are expressed. When we think of our own lives we can think of recurrent themes or patterns which manifest themselves in quite different ways at different times, although the theme remains the same. Then I came across a phrase in Kelly's writings which said that elements change but constructs often remain the same. Kelly's ideas came together with my previous ideas about themes.

Windy Dryden: Once you had identified important themes with these patients how did you then attempt to deal with them?

Don Bannister: What we would do now was really two things. First we could actually begin to talk and the interesting thing here was that the talk seemed far less circular and far more like what you hope your communication with patients in psychotherapy will be like. What did surprise me was the rapidity with which, once I felt that I had somehow arrived at some things approximating the theme, the delusional trimmings were dropped. Sometimes that effect was quite startling. Quite often it didn't have to be a very subtle guess if you see what I mean. It could be a broad one. It is not uncommon with so-called psychotics to get various forms of delusion about sexual anatomy and process. One common delusion, that I have encountered several times, concerns the person believing that his sperm is accumulating and will shortly choke him. Now if you simply start the conversation on the general line that sex has always been a difficult area for them, you seem to be into the topic fairly rapidly without making any very brilliant psychoanalytic insights about early traumas. It is picking out the theme. I am saying something not much cleverer than: 'If you have got these anatomical ideas about sexual processes then you probably are bothered by sex, fearful of its threats and dangers. So let's talk about that.'

Windy Dryden: So, what you are saying is that, first and foremost, the identification of the the theme enabled you to actually establish more of a therapeutic alliance with the patient and enable you to start to deal with their concerns?

Don Bannister: Yes, 'dealing' with also included the fact that I could now begin to work on devising practical exercises or experiments with clients. I was more able to work within a construct theory mode where therapy consists of a cyclic alternation between reflection and exploration, reconstruing and trying out the new construing in practice. In other words, when you do certain things, seeing if what happens is what you anticipated happening, on the basis of your interpretation of the situation. So it is really a cycling between the theory and the experiment. So I was now able to work with the so-called psychotic to set up lines of practical exploration.

Coming back to the case of the young man I mentioned earlier the interesting thing was that it turned out to be possible to get him to go and talk to three doctors about their attitude to him. He remained convinced that two of them were hostile to him but he managed to form some kind of relationship with the third doctor. We were then able to arrange that this man should be his doctor—all without reference to the lorries. The interesting thing was that at this stage he did not want to bring the lorries into conversations. I had warned the doctor that he was able to form some relationship with (to whom he had now been assigned) that if lorries came into the conversation, he was to stick to the general theme of their relationship. However the lorries rarely came into the picture. So it did prove possible to develop testable notions and to get some kind of exploration going.

Windy Dryden: So are you saying that once you have not been distracted by the delusional talk, you can use it as a point of entry, by identifying themes, to work in a way that would be similar to therapy with neurotic patients?

Don Bannister: Yes, it wouldn't be basically different, although working with so-called psychotics is a longer enterprise by quite a bit. You can think in terms of years rather than months quite often. It has differences of that kind but basically I don't think that it is a different kind of undertaking, particularly if you give it enough time. It has got to have time to work its way through. My impression now is that the delusions that are offered serve certain purposes. One is that they do actually contain the concern of the client which is why it is worth trying to work out what the theme is. The delusions are not arbitrary, whimsical or nonsensical. They contain a story, and embedded in that story is the client's concern. Another purpose served by the delusions is that they help such clients to maintain distance between themselves and other people and certainly delusions are highly successful ways of maintaining distance. Certainly, my impression is that most so-called psychotics have an enormous distrust of people. Sometimes I wonder whether the delusions not only maintain a barrier but also act as a kind of test and only people who are prepared to somehow come through the delusions would be, to any degree, trusted. This impression is still quite tentative, but I sometimes get the feeling that the client begins to trust me after we have explored and somehow got through the delusion. However, it is interesting that trust goes on being tested time and time again, which is incidentally part of the reason why therapy takes much longer with so-called psychotics. So-called neurotics will often trust the therapy relationship after a relatively short time and work on that basis. However, most psychotic patients are not going to trust the therapist for quite a long time and they are going to do a lot of testing before they will place trust in the therapist.

Windy Dryden: So, it sounds as if you have come to see the formation of delusional symptons as reflecting another kind of theme concerning their difficulties trusting and getting close to people. This is very different from the more traditional viewpoint which states that these symptons can be attributed to biochemical disturbances of one sort or another.

Don Bannister: Yes, but then I never quite see how biochemical disturbance can produce a way of thinking. You know how some people giggle when you are teaching the history of psychology and you come to the bit where Descartes believed that the seat of the soul is the pineal gland. Now if you are going to giggle at that view, I think you should giggle too at the thought that it is purines in the urine or taraxin or some biochemical that produces schizophrenia.

Windy Dryden: Have you spent much time speculating about the origins of these symptoms?

Don Bannister: Yes. I think the interesting thing is the more you come to know so-called psychotics, the more intelligible their experience becomes. You find in the long run that so-called psychosis is no more profoundly puzzling than so-called neurosis. In fact it is like a neurosis, only if you like the journey has gone further. I take the view that there is no dualism here. There are not two kinds of complaints. I would be inclined to say that if you push the neurotic journey far enough then people will start to call you psychotic. However, it is our labelling that is different. Interestingly enough, the main reason for the addition of the label psychotic is the question of delusions. When talk becomes bizarre and incomprehensible, that's the point at which we start to talk about madness or psychosis as opposed to neurosis rather than because behaviour has become all that much more bizarre. I think we are very much influenced by communication. If we can't talk to someone, we become very disturbed by them.

Windy Dryden: You mentioned in your letter to me about this project that although you did eventually take up a particular stance, which we have discussed, you still feel somewhat in a dilemma about this issue. I wonder if you could articulate what remains of the dilemma for you?

Don Bannister: What remains a dilemma is that I still find myself, at times, unwilling to try to understand, highlight and follow through on the underlying theme. I find that, even after all this time, I can still become very angry with delusional talk and suddenly break into arguing with it and for a period I say to myself, 'I won't stand this nonsense any more. I will not have this kind of crap poured on my head,' and I become angry and try to rebut their delusions and I tend to shout a bit. Or at other times I find myself dropping back to humouring again. What remains of my dilemma is that I still cannot *easily* or *readily* accept delusional talk. However much I convince myself that there is a way through it and that it makes a kind of sense if we can get at the themes, there is something about delusional talk which I still find disturbing, anger-provoking, or at least irritating. That doesn't seem to be something I can ever quite get out of. It's an effort all of the time.

Windy Dryden: I think there is some early literature that suggested that certain types of therapist were more comfortable in dealing with so-called psychotic patients than so-called neurotic patients. You seem to be basically comfortable in working with psychotic patients but what you are saying is that you have limits.

Don Bannister: Yes, there are limits to working with anybody on God's earth. There are people one ultimately can't cope with, quite outside the context of therapy. But yes, I think, strangely enough that what my residual anger is about or what my difficulty with it is, is because it is *talk*. The person pretends to communicate and yet does not communicate. What is at issue between you and the psychotic is that the psychotic is *apparently* communicating, explaining, offering you something in the way of talk and yet what you get is something that is not communication, something simply baffling or frightening. I say this because I have worked with a lot of psychotics and I am rarely ever upset by their behaviour. Psychotics do strange things at times, they will throw things about or stand on their heads or get in bed and pull the sheets over them so you have to speak to them through the sheets for hours or they will shit on the floor. They will do all kinds of strange things but somehow I don't find that such behaviour worries me greatly. I am upset by it, sometimes. However I can respond to it or I can accept it because in a sense there is no pretence about it. It is the way they want to behave. But when they talk to me it is like . . . I say to you, talk to me and then you pretend to talk to me but you are not talking to me.

Windy Dryden: It's the pretence which you are angry about? And that's your particular limitation?

Don Bannister: Yes, it is. In a way I know it's foolish because I know from experience that if I work with it I will get through. But it still feels as if the psychotic has broken part of the contract we had between us. I think there is an unwritten contract between people, an agreement to try to explain their feelings and desires to each other and to try to do that to the best of their ability. The psychotic has secretly torn up that contract. It is when this contract is not fulfilled that I am faced with my own limitations.

Windy Dryden: Well, I think you have actually fulfilled your contract with me. Thank you very much.

DISCUSSION ISSUES

1. *Do you consider that 'psychosis' is due to 'biochemical disturbances of one sort or another'? If not, what factors do you consider are involved?*
2. *Do you believe that it is possible to do productive psychotherapy with 'psychotic' clients? If so, what form might such therapy take?*
3. *How do you respond in therapy to a 'psychotic' client's delusional talk?*
4. *Are you more personally disturbed by 'psychotics'' delusional talk or by their bizarre behaviour? Why?*
5. *What clients do you personally find it difficult to work with in therapy and why?*

CHAPTER SIXTEEN

Therapists' Dilemmas as Stimuli to New Understanding and Practice

Tim Bond

This book opened with the observation that therapists' dilemmas are seldom aired in public, either in publications or at conferences except during late night discussions. The foregoing collection of therapists' dilemmas posed by eminent and experienced therapists begs the question of whether therapists' dilemmas deserve to be shunned. What is being avoided by remaining silent about these dilemmas?

A partial response can be found in the generally negative construction placed on the concept of a dilemma. Dictionary definitions focus almost exclusively on their adverse features. For example, the *New Shorter Oxford Dictionary* defines dilemma as 'A choice between two (or several) alternatives which are equally unfavourable; a position of doubt or perplexity; a difficult situation' (Brown, 1993). If this is the comprehensive encapsulation of a dilemma, then little wonder they are shunned in public disclosure. To admit to a dilemma is to be personally vulnerable to an emotional sense of being pulled in two directions at once, in combination with considerable cognitive uncertainty. A public admission of a dilemma may also be viewed as challenging the profession's image of competence and reliability of service and could therefore be construed as undermining of the individual and collective self interest of therapists. Fortunately, this is not the whole story. The existence of these interviews and the apparent willingness of the interviewees to participate in a public airing of their dilemmas as therapists suggests that there may also be, although until now unnoticed, positive features to discussing dilemmas. In this chapter I shall analyse some features of the interviews to extrapolate the interviewee's experience of their dilemmas, giving attention both to negative and to positive aspects of their dilemmas. In any form of analysis it is always worth considering what has been omitted which might be significant in the total picture. One category of therapists' dilemmas is totally absent and I shall begin with these because they demonstrate the destructive potential of some dilemmas.

DILEMMAS WHICH UNDERMINE THE THERAPIST'S MOTIVATION

A characteristic shared by all the therapists interviewed in this book is their commitment to continuing to provide therapy. None of the dilemmas presented are of a kind which has substantially shaken that commitment. However, in my experience as a trainer, and occasionally as a counsellor of therapists, I have encountered people experiencing dilemmas which lead them actively to question their continuing commitment to provide therapy and in some cases, as a result, temporarily or permanently abandoning their role as therapist. For example, therapists known to me have temporarily withdrawn from their work and re-evaluated their role as therapist following, variously, separation from their partner, bereavement, or the birth of a disabled child.

Dilemmas which can undermine someone's motivation as a therapist appear to arise in three broad categories. Some people discover an area of personal vulnerability which is so painful that their energy is directed towards self-protection or self-healing to such an extent that they are no longer able to perceive or respond to their clients' needs. Paradoxically, there is also the opposite extreme: some people grow out of a personal need which was satisfied by being a therapist, so the motivation disappears, and they move on to more personally satisfying work. These situations being so personal and individual it is unsurprising that they barely feature in the public discourse of the profession: one group may feel too vulnerable to share their experience in public; the other has diverted their attention elsewhere.

A third category are those therapists who become seriously disillusioned either with therapy as an activity, or with therapists collectively as represented by their profession. That personal accounts of this kind of disillusionment are so rare is surprising. Those who leave the profession of therapy usually do so quietly. Jeffrey Masson is a notable exception. In *Final Analysis* (1990), Masson describes his disenchantment with psychoanalysis as a result of personal experience and intellectual questioning, which led him finally to abandon his work as a therapist. One of his doubts concerned the intellectual honesty of Sigmund Freud as the founder of therapy. Masson grew to dislike the collective culture of the eminent psychoanalysts he encountered, finding them emotionally distant and lacking in personal openness. He was also frequently bored when providing therapy. The combined effect of these and other considerations made Masson's resolution of his dilemma about whether to remain a therapist almost inevitable. Arguably, the public airing of the dilemma, and his critique of psycho-analysis, is beneficial both to those who share his predicament and to those of us who remain committed to therapy. Masson's account of his own experience affirms his commitment to truth and personal integrity, and thereby challenges our own commitment to these values.

Although the dilemmas raised by the therapists in this book are not of a kind which overwhelm the interviewee's commitment to being a therapist, they share some of the positive values espoused by Masson. They represent a commitment to truth in exploring the implications for therapy of a particular dilemma and what it reveals about the limitations of therapy. During the interview with Arnold Lazarus there is a good example of questioning established practice: '. . . at least 90 per cent of resistance is due to therapist ignorance' (page 164). Instead of being demotivated by this knowledge, Lazarus commits himself to attempting to provide a more adequate understanding of the nature of resistance in order to be of greater assistance to clients. The clear expression of the dilemma represents a personal acknowledgement of what may well be a significant limitation of therapy, but it does not undermine the whole enterprise. I shall return to this point later when I consider the challenge that therapists' dilemmas pose to the profession. Next, however, I want to explore the implications of therapists' dilemmas for work with current clients.

THE CHALLENGE OF DILEMMAS IN A CURRENT THERAPEUTIC RELATIONSHIP

The dilemmas posed in this book, whilst not of the kind to undermine the therapist's motivation to remaining a therapist, could have profound implications for any current client. The existence of a dilemma is already indicative of a potential threat to the therapeutic relationship because there is no way forward without the risk of encountering the disadvantages of any of the available options. For example, to trust the autonomy of a suicidal client risks the client's life, but to breach confidentiality to obtain assistance for the client risks the therapeutic relationship. The dilemma would disappear if an unproblematic option became apparent, if, for example, the client ceased to be suicidal or actively wanted additional assistance. The persistence of the dilemma represents a challenge to the therapist's management of the immediate situation within a given therapeutic relationship. The therapist is under pressure to resolve the dilemma and/or to mitigate potential harm to the client. An inappropriate choice of the available options could harm the therapeutic work, either temporarily by disrupting it, or, by prompting the client to abandon therapy. Some inappropriate responses to the dilemma might actively harm the client.

Several of the interviewees recognized the potential for harm as a constraint on their options for resolving a dilemma. Paul Watchel rejected certain ways of challenging a 'non-improving patient' as being too brutal and hurtful, or, at the other extreme, ineffective (page 145). He was seeking a balance between listening and therapeutic zeal (page 148). The choice between offering a client the comfort of personal warmth or the discomfort of therapeutic challenge also preoccupied Albert Ellis. These dilemmas demand actual decisions in the management of particular clients. There is sometimes enough leeway for the therapist to consider the options: at worst, a client remaining stuck during the decision-making process. In other circumstances, however, time to ponder may be in short supply: there is an urgency when resolving dilemmas when working with a client who is starving to death. This was the dilemma posed by Fay Fransella, in which the risk to the client was a good deal more serious than merely prolonging a period of non-improvement. The imminent danger was physical deterioration, irreversible damage, and even death.

Most experienced therapists have encountered in their practice dilemmas requiring urgent resolution. How the interviewees in this book responded to their dilemmas shows us an interesting range of possible responses, which include:

(a) Choosing one of the available options   Marcia Davis was faced with sharing or withholding her case notes from a client who had become unproductively preoccupied with what she was recording about him. She resolved

the dilemma by showing the notes to her client whilst being mindful of the dangers in doing so both to herself (of being excessively self-revealing) and to the client (of being too critical or too negative about him). She made her decision after reading the notes that she had written and therefore was able to make an assessment of the potential for harm in comparison with the potential for benefit. In this way she sought to mitigate the negative aspects of this option. With the benefit of her experience behind her, she revised some aspects of her note taking in order to free herself to share her notes with other clients. In pursuing one option, she actively sought to mitigate its potential for harm with the current client and took preventive action to avoid a recurrence of the dilemma for future clients.

(b) Taking a middle route between the horns of the dilemma John Bancroft preferred to consider himself an educator, a role which he viewed as more facilitative than that of a healer which he perceived as more authoritative and akin to his role as a doctor. In his work as a sex therapist he often experienced a dilemma of feeling under pressure to move from being an educator to becoming a healer in order to meet the client's expectations or needs. He resolved the dilemma by adopting a middle route in which he avoids extended assessment procedures which might encourage dependence on his expertise rather than clients taking responsibility for themselves. Whilst he permits himself to be directive in terms of recommending certain programmes of activity, he does so in a way which invites clients to share their reflections and personal learning as a result of participating in the programme. In this way he attempts to provide a sense of direction and purpose without becoming prescriptive or ignoring the client's responsibility for their own progress. He has defined for himself a middle course which avoids the least desirable aspects of the options which constitute the dilemma.

(c) Sharing responsibility with the client for resolving the dilemma Peter Lomas presents the dilemma of the influence of the therapist's moral values on the client. He does not accept that one can be a neutral facilitator and even if it were possible it would be immoral to remain neutral (page 99). He finally resolved his dilemma by being explicit about his own morals in a way which was sensitive to the client's circumstances with a view to encouraging open discussion between the therapist and client. Thus he avoided, and indeed minimized the risk of, imposing his values on the client, and he also avoided creating a false impression of moral neutrality. This willingness to involve the client in resolving the dilemma would not

suit all situations or all the therapists. Fay Fransella doubted the usefulness of sharing her dilemma with a teenager who was starving herself to death (page 133). Similarly Dougal McKay rejected the option of sharing his dilemma with someone who was suicidal (page 122). In these circumstances, the therapists considered that it was their sole responsibility to manage the dilemma.

(d) Avoidance of the dilemma   Once a dilemma has been identified it might be possible to avoid it either by referring a current client to another source of help or by avoiding taking on any client likely to raise the dilemma. Fay Fransella reflects that, by asking a colleague to undertake the work, she sidesteps her dilemma between following Kelly's principles, which she considers essential to her way of working, and the requirements for acting against the client's wishes when working with severe eating disorders (page 132).

(e) Progressive refinement of responses to the dilemma   Don Bannister has never totally resolved his area of discomfort in working with psychotics, but by progressively trying a number of strategies and reflecting on the experience, he has found an optimal strategy which also clarifies his area of unease. The dilemma was not extinguished, but its negative impact was considerably curtailed for him as a therapist and the possibility of therapeutic progress for the client was considerably enhanced (page 178).

(f) 'Watchful waiting'   No one explicitly refers to maintaining a state of watchful waiting but this appears to be the strategy adopted by Arnold Lazarus with a patient who is unable to progress and who might be considered 'resistant' in other approaches to therapy. He is looking actively for clues about what maintains the client in a seemingly stable position both when he was with the client, and independently of his client work in his research. When faced with any of a combination of inadequate knowledge of the client's situation, inadequate professional theory and an absence of any proven strategy, a state of active watchfulness seems a sensible and humane response.

   In Britain, most therapists and counsellors raise issues over the management of their clients within a supervisory relationship. Regular and ongoing supervision is an ethical requirement for counsellors (BAC, 1993: B.3.1), counselling psychologists (BPS, 1995: 2.1.2) but it is not a universal requirement for registered psychotherapists (UKCP, 1995). Even when it is not a strict requirement, anecdotal evidence suggests that most therapists use some form of confidential consultation with an experienced colleague to talk through these dilemmas as they relate to the management of their clients. The theory and practice of supervision is rapidly becoming a discipline in its own right (Foskett and Lyall, 1988; Proctor, 1988; Hawkins and Shohet, 1989; Feltham and Dryden, 1994; Page and Woskett, 1994; Carroll, 1996).

In many ways the interviews conducted by Windy Dryden have some of the characteristics of a supervisory session. The therapist is facilitated to explore the dilemma from several angles. These include giving attention to standards, openness to new learning and development, and personal support, which are respectively supervisory tasks identified by Proctor (1988) as normative, formative and supportive. However, there are also features in the interviews which may be less typical of supervision as it is currently practised and yet they allow the therapist to discuss aspects of their work in a meaningful and enlightening way. As experienced practitioners, and perhaps because of the public nature of the interview, the interviewees were not looking for specific resolutions to dilemmas in particular cases. Presumably, to have done so would have compromised their clients' confidentiality. Instead, most of each interview was an opportunity to take an overview of an important or recurrent dilemma independently of the context of specific cases (except for illustrative purposes). The reader is the main beneficiary of this approach because it sets the dilemma in a general context. However, there are also gains to the therapist and to the profession. I will consider each of these in turn. Partly in response to careful consideration of these interviews, and also as a result of other research I have conducted (Bond, 1991), I think there is a strong case for widening the scope of supervision, so that supervisors provide opportunities to take an overview of patterns in the therapeutic work of their supervisees, including recurrent dilemmas and contextual issues. Dilemmas challenge not only our direct work with clients, but perhaps also our sense of ourselves, and the organization of our profession.

THE PERSONALLY REFLEXIVE CHALLENGE OF DILEMMAS

Each of the interviews offers the reader an insight into the person being interviewed. In many cases it is unclear whether the interviewee is sharing familiar material about themselves and their work or whether they have gained some personal insight as a result of the interview. However, one interview stands out as generating new personal insights for the interviewee. Paul Brown's reflections on when to make scientific or therapeutic interventions leads him to realize that the dilemma occurs in an acute form only when the scientific observation is apparently painful to the client or when the client is pessimistic about the future (page 112).

Several therapists raise the recurrent dilemma of when to give power to the client and when the therapist ought to exercise power in the interests of the client. They raise the dilemma in many guises: as a choice between scientific and therapeutic interventions (Lazarus and Brown), therapeutic challenge or warmth (Ellis), listening or therapeutic zeal (Watchel), and confrontation or collusion (Mackay). I was left wondering about whether these formulations of what appears to be the therapists' perennial dilemma are revealing of the therapists as people. Whilst any answer from these interviews remains speculative, clues in the personal preoccupations and style of speech suggest that it is a question worth asking within supervision. There may be a reflexive relationship between the dilemma that someone presents and their sense of themselves, which may be tacit or readily accessible to the interviewee. My own reflections have encouraged me to consider the possibility of generating new insights into myself by considering the dilemmas which I regularly present in supervision as a source of reflexive learning. Is it possible the dilemma is an outward manifestation of an internal split within my sense of self? For example, some years ago I was working with several couples in which one person wished to sustain the relationship but the other wanted separation from what they experienced as a highly demanding and dependent partner. As a counsellor I actively facilitated the discussion between the partners but in supervision I expressed an unusual depth of personal conflict about the best way forward. Initially I talked about what had become a painful dilemma in working with one couple. Then I realized this was a theme which ran through my presentations of several cases and that I was the common factor, not the clients or their difficulties. This was the first step of starting to face up to being in a relationship which was becoming intolerable to me.

One of the characteristics of dilemmas is to challenge any personal pretensions towards omniscience or omnipotence. Don Bannister confronts this issue directly and succinctly. After describing how he had improved his way of responding to psychotic talking, he explained that this had not totally resolved the dilemma. He is still left with a feeling that a psychotic patient has secretly torn up the 'unwritten contract between people, an agreement to try to explain their feelings and desires to each other. . . . It is when this contract is not fulfilled that I am faced with my own limitations' (page 178). Acknowledgement of dilemmas highlighting personal limitations is implicit in other interviews.

DILEMMAS AS A CHALLENGE TO THERAPY AS A PROFESSION

It is well known that therapy can be too self-referential at the expense of awareness of social structures. It is also possible that the source of the dilemma may not rest in the therapist as individual but in the collective construction of therapy as a profession. The main focus of some dilemmas challenges current professional structures and systems. Some dilemmas are presented as an individual attempting to find an appropriate place for themselves within the structure of the profession. Richard Wessler speaks movingly of the price he paid for leaving his post at the Institute of RET in New York in order to maintain his sense of integrity about the model of therapy he practised (page 86). Painful though this change was, it resolved his dilemma.

Other dilemmas demand less drastic action but challenge an established corpus of professional knowledge. As a leading cognitive behaviourist, Marvin Goldfried challenges the usual practice of concentrating on the client's current life situation outside the therapy session rather than on problems which emerge within the therapy session. He describes a number of instances which therapists with a psychodynamic orientation would identify as transference, a terminology and conceptual framework which seems incompatible with a cognitive behavioural orientation. He resolved the dilemma by expanding the data he is willing to attend to as a therapist and referring to those elements in the theory of transference which are most compatible with his core model. In this instance, the dilemma has been a stimulus to change in the body of knowledge. Arnold Lazarus offers a similar challenge to the concept of resistance. Resolving dilemmas by drawing on the theory and practice of other therapeutic approaches is so widespread that a vigorous debate about syncretism, eclecticism and integration has been stimulated (Norcross and Tomcho, 1993). Dilemmas may be indicative of the limitations of current knowledge as well as prompts to new developments.

It is characteristic of a profession to seek to identify the activities which fall within its scope and as a consequence certain boundaries in practice are established.

Brian Thorne's dilemma led him to question the extent to which effective counselling can be restricted to one-hour sessions within the counselling room and whether what might usually be considered social contact has a positive benefit. Such considerations often fall within the scope of professional ethics, usually as dual relationships (Bond, 1993). Paul Watchel pointed out that the boundary between therapeutic decisions and ethics is not clearly defined. Even working within the accepted boundaries, a therapist may experience conflicting responsibilities which have an ethical dimension (page 145).

Many of the dilemmas presented in this book can be reframed as pointing to limitations in the present knowledge and organizational systems which constitute therapy. The dilemmas challenge all therapists to recognize their collective limitations and may point to possible areas for future developments.

THE CHALLENGE OF THERAPISTS' DILEMMAS

I started with the negative aspects of the dilemmas. There can be no denying that dilemmas are intrinsically uncomfortable experiences. They discomfort us by throwing us into a quandary of difficult choices in situations where there are no obviously solely beneficial options, and all options have significant disadvantages. However, I hope that this analysis of some aspects of the interviews has challenged the view that dilemmas are invariably negative, characterized by emotional pain and cognitive uncertainty. The collective responses of the therapists interviewed in this book suggests that this is only a, partial picture of dilemmas. Dilemmas may well combine some dysfunctional with some functional capabilities. When they arise, dilemmas pose immediate challenges regarding work with a current client, which frequently tests therapist, client and the therapist's supervisor. Outside the immediate therapeutic relationship, dilemmas can be seen to act as boundary markers of the competence of the individual therapist and the profession as a whole. Dilemmas chase us away from a tendency to see ourselves as omnipotent and omniscient. They do not necessarily undermine the value and purpose of therapy. It seems a pity that such a rich vein in the therapist's experience is so seldom mined for what it reveals about us as therapists. Windy Dryden is to be congratulated in being the first to draw together such a collection. The participating therapists are also to be applauded for breaking the silence in print about therapists' dilemmas.

I anticipate that most therapists would agree with Paul Watchel '. . . doing therapy inevitably involves dilemmas. There is no way to avoid dilemmas. The best we can do is to mitigate them and help to make them constructive experiences' (page 144). Part of the transformation of dilemmas into constructive experiences is not simply racing to resolve them, even were this possible; it is to rise to the challenge of learning from the dilemma about what its existence tells us about our own involvement in the provision of therapy, and about the nature of therapy itself.

REFERENCES

Bond, T. (1991). *HIV Counselling: Report of National Survey and Consultation*. Rugby: British Association for Counselling.

Bond, T. (1993). *Standards and Ethics for Counsellors in Action*. London: Sage.

British Association for Counselling (BAC) (1993). *Code of Ethics and Practice for Counsellors*. Rugby: British Association for Counselling.

British Psychological Society (BPS) (1995). *Guidelines for the Professional Practice of Counselling Psychology*. Leicester: British Psychological Society.

Brown, L. (ed.) (1993). *The New Shorter Oxford English Dictionary*. Oxford: Clarendon Press.

Carroll, M. (1996). *Counselling Supervision: Theory, Skills and Practice*. London: Cassell.

Feltham, C. and Dryden, W. (1994). *Developing Counselling Supervision*. London: Sage.

Foskett, J. and Lyall, D. (1988). *Helping the Helpers – Supervision and Pastoral Care*. London: SPCK.

Hawkins, P. and Shohet, R. (1989). *Supervision in the Helping Professions*. Buckingham: Open University Press.

Masson, J. (1990). *Final Analysis – The Making and Unmaking of a Psychoanalyst*. London: HarperCollins.

Norcross, J.C. and Tomcho, T.J. (1993). 'Choosing an eclectic, not syncretic, psychotherapist' in W. Dryden (ed.) *Questions and Answers on Counselling in Action*. London: Sage. pp 81–5.

Page, S. and Woskett, V. (1994). *Supervising the Counsellor – a Cyclical Model*. London: Routledge.

Proctor, B. (1988). 'Supervision: a co-operative exercise in accountability' in M. Marken and M. Payne (eds) *Enabling and Ensuring Supervision in Practice*. Leicester: National Youth Bureau. pp. 21–34.

United Kingdom Council for Psychotherapy (UKCP) (1995). *Ethical Guidelines*. London: United Kingdom Council for Psychotherapy.

INDEX OF NAMES

193

INDEX OF SUBJECTS

Index compiled by Peva Keane